Book Description

Men over 50 are a demographic that tends to be forgotten when it comes to health and wellness, but there has been a significant increase in understanding how our nutritional needs change as we age. The Mediterranean Diet is a catch-all term for the diet of nations along the Mediterranean Sea. It emphasises wholegrains, includes plenty of fruits and vegetables, has room for poultry and lots of oily fish, and allows a moderate intake of red wine if that's your thing. While this diet is no miracle pill that will help you lose weight, you do stand to gain a lot of health benefits from following it! The Mediterranean Diet is easy to follow and can help to improve your general health and wellbeing.

This book covers a general introduction to the diet, including advice regarding intermittent fasting and sample recipes for your personal use. You will also find some general advice on different types of exercise that you may or may not want to implement in your daily life. Most of what you will find between these pages comes from a mix of personal experience following the diet and research into its benefits. Before we get into it, there are a couple of general 'rules' to follow when preparing your meals. Around half of your plate should consist of non-starchy vegetables, a quarter should be healthy proteins, and the remaining quarter should be wholegrains. The main thing is you get it all in your diet!

The Mediterranean Diet For Men Over 50

Intermittent Fasting, Recipes, A Little History, Exercise, And Advice!

Patrick Thompson

© Copyright 2021 - All rights reserved.

The content contained within this book may not be reproduced, duplicated or transmitted without direct written permission from the author or the publisher.

Under no circumstances will any blame or legal responsibility be held against the publisher, or author, for any damages, reparation, or monetary loss due to the information contained within this book, either directly or indirectly.

Legal Notice:

This book is copyright protected. It is only for personal use. You cannot amend, distribute, sell, use, quote or paraphrase any part, or the content within this book, without the consent of the author or publisher.

Disclaimer Notice:

Please note the information contained within this document is for educational and entertainment purposes only. All effort has been executed to present accurate, up to date, reliable, complete information. No warranties of any kind are declared or implied. Readers acknowledge that the author is not engaged in the rendering of legal, financial, medical or professional advice. The content within this book has been derived from various sources. Please consult a licensed professional before attempting any techniques outlined in this book.

By reading this document, the reader agrees that under no circumstances is the author responsible for any losses, direct or indirect, that are incurred as a result of the use of the information contained within this document, including, but not limited to, errors, omissions, or inaccuracies.

Table of Contents

Book Description
Table of Contents
Introduction
Chapter 1: The Mediterranean Diet
  The Mediterranean Diet: A History
    Modern Components Of The Diet
Chapter 2: Benefits
  Nutrition
  The Pros
    ... And A Few Cons
    Conclusion
Chapter 3: Recipes
    Breakfast
    Lunch
    Dinner
    Sweets And Puddings
    Snacks
    Conclusion
Chapter 4: Things To Expect When You Change Diets
Chapter 5: Intermittent Fasting
  What To Expect When You Start Intermittent Fasting
    The Benefits Of Intermittent Fasting
    Conclusion

Chapter 6: Get Moving!
   Some Great Ways To Move
      Yoga
      HIIT
      Weight Training
      Cycling And Spinning
      Swimming
      Bodyweight Exercise
      Cardio
      Running
      Walking
      General Activity
      A Note On Safety
      Conclusion
Conclusion
References

Introduction

I love food. Who doesn't? Enjoying a good meal with your family is one of life's little pleasures, but indulging a bit too much can cause some trouble. When I was (much!) younger, I struggled a lot with my weight, constantly trying the latest fad diet. Everything from protein shakes only to excessive calorie cutting. Just jumping from one diet to the next, thinking it would help. It's true what they say about yo-yo dieting: you always regain the weight you lose, sometimes with interest. What I found was that the companies selling the latest quick-fix weight-loss shake or supplement were not at all interested in helping me lose weight. It was, literally, all about the sale. What made it worse was that I was *active*. Surely, I thought, being active would help me shift the pounds and stones?

Nope. Being active is an important part of weight loss and maintaining health, but what we eat is just as important. Just over 21 years ago, I lost my mother, and it was a bit of a wake-up call. I decided to make a series of changes to my diet. I cut out refined carbohydrates, included more oils and healthy fats, upped my intake of fruits and vegetables, and made a point of getting a good walk in as well as getting some high-powered workouts in. When I made these changes, my health improved dramatically. I felt better than I ever had when I was yo-yo dieting. At first, I thought I was on the keto diet because I was getting in more healthy proteins, but when I actually looked at what keto is—a diet that emphasises high fat intake and moderate protein intake with few carbohydrates—I realised that that could not be it. It turned out that I was following a Mediterranean Diet!

Following this diet has really helped me understand what goes into making a healthy lifestyle. One example I can give you is that your weight isn't just about how much fat there is on your body. A kilogram of muscle is denser than a kilogram of fat, so when you exercise, it should be with the intention of burning fat and improving your overall strength.

Another thing is that restriction diets, like those fad milkshake ones, are determined to tell you that you *absolutely are not* allowed to treat yourself. There's plenty of evidence that restricting yourself and denying yourself the treats you love will only lead to a relapse. Because you go so long without it, you overindulge when you 'allow' yourself to have it 'just once.'

Something else I've learned is that no food is inherently 'good' or 'bad.' All food is just fuel for the body, and it's perfectly fine to just enjoy it. The Mediterranean Diet is full of flavour, rich in a diversity of foods, and has no restrictions. You just need to be mindful about what you eat and how much. It's probably the most common-sense way of eating I've come across in all my years.

Broadly speaking, 'Mediterranean Diet' is a catch-all term for the national diets found in countries along the Mediterranean. If you were in Italy or France or Spain, you might just consider it your daily diet. In the UK, the diet generally consists of fruits and vegetables, and plenty of whole grains and healthy fats. You're probably thinking, 'this sounds like a vegetarian diet,' and I can see why you might think that. It's probably closer to a flexitarian model because you have a bit of room to add fish and poultry. There's not that much room for red meat, so a weekly treat could be your Sunday roast! You have plenty of opportunities to include protein on this diet if you don't feel like including fish and poultry. You can enjoy a moderate intake of beans and eggs. However, if you're like I used to be and really love your cheese, it's going to be a struggle for you to limit your intake. Again, it's all about moderation. Don't overindulge. Have some mozzarella melted over a nice thick slice of sourdough with some olive oil and a bit of crushed garlic, or a scoop of low-fat probiotic yoghurt with some fruit, and your dairy cravings will be satiated.

This book exists because men over 50 are so often ignored when it comes to health and wellness. Plenty of books exist for young men, young women, and women over 50. There are even videos on YouTube explaining why certain fad diets are perfect for specific age groups! But there are limited options for men over 50. Anyone can benefit from eating a Mediterranean Diet, although my goal for this book is to help men in my age group understand how they can benefit. You might not want to lose weight. You might just want to feel healthier. You might have a medication that requires you to have a certain amount of oil every day. Or you might want to completely overhaul your eating habits and get healthier. Whatever your personal situation, I encourage you to give the Mediterranean Diet a go.

In this book, I am going to take you through not only the diet but also intermittent fasting, a few recipes, and a sample exercise plan. Intermittent fasting is an eating schedule that includes extended periods of abstaining from food. Some of the types of fasting are quite common sense, while others are a bit more awkward to implement. The recipes included in the book are a mix of breakfast, lunch, and dinner options with a couple of pudding options. Yes, you can enjoy sweet treats while following the Mediterranean Diet!

Notice how I'm not referring to the Mediterranean Diet as a diet in the sense of 'this will help you lose weight.' That is because, in its simplest form, diet consists of food that people habitually eat. A national diet could center on meat and starchy vegetables, like the British diet, or it could be full of healthy vegetables and oils, like the Mediterranean Diet. Medical diets also exist which often take the form of a short-term course. The ketogenic diet started out this way, as a prescribed diet for children who suffer from epilepsy. However, as the name implies, medical diets should be done under medical supervision. As the health and wellness industry has grown, it has appropriated the term 'diet,' and a variety of fad diets have grown out of it. Fad diets are diets that become popular for short periods of time but are generally not sustainable. These diets typically involve cutting out or restricting certain foods. The Mediterranean Diet differs because it actually *is* sustainable and does not involve cutting things out. I will say again: it's all about moderation.

By the time you finish this book, I want you to have a better understanding of what the Mediterranean Diet looks like and how you might be able to implement it in your daily life. You do not need to live in Italy or Greece to enjoy it. You simply need to be open to trying new foods and getting to know the fuel you're giving your body. It can be quite difficult to implement, especially if you are new to cooking. Most of the meals you will be eating should be cooked from scratch, although there is plenty of room for getting your meals ready ahead of time. Now, I think we should begin by taking a thorough, in-depth look at what the Mediterranean Diet is.

Chapter 1: The Mediterranean Diet

In simple terms, the Mediterranean Diet is a collection of diets followed by countries that border the Mediterranean Sea. These countries are typically in the 'olive-growing' region, most notably Italy and Greece, although Spain and France have their own versions of the diet. 'Mediterranean' can be viewed as an umbrella term in this context. For this reason, the Mediterranean Diet is perhaps the most varied diet option out there. It doesn't cut out your favorite foods, but it adds a whole bunch of new sources of vitamins and minerals. You can also adapt it to fit your personal needs. The ketogenic diet, for example, can easily be made a bit more Mediterranean if you adjust your macros properly. Vegetarians and vegans can also benefit from the rich variety of oils and nutrient-dense vegetables in this diet.

As the Mediterranean Diet has grown in popularity, it has gained a reputation as yet another 'trendy diet.' The reason behind this is the influence of celebrity culture, although this has long since faded into obscurity. For months, cookbooks filled with 'Greek-style' and 'Italian-inspired' recipes filled the shelves at bookstores across Europe and the United States. Cooking shows that featured hearty recipes of fish, lean meats, and pasta dominated the airwaves in the early 2010s. Then, it faded. But the influence of these cookbooks remains strong. Now, the Mediterranean Diet is experiencing something of a rebirth.

Any diet has its pros and cons, and in a later chapter, we will address the pros and cons of the Mediterranean Diet. For now, I want to give you a brief history of the diet, an overview of what it is, and how you can expect to benefit from it.

The Mediterranean Diet: A History

The history of diet is long, varied, and interesting, but one thing remains consistent: the diet is shaped by its people and their will to survive. Research into early man often focuses on the 'hunter gatherers' who subsisted mainly on nuts and berries foraged from nearby sources, while hunters fought to bring down big game. These actions fed into the desire to survive, which eventually evolved into farming. Farming can be traced back to roughly 10 000 BC and the rest, as they say, is history. Humans developed and passed down agricultural knowledge, which today is worth around 25% of the global economy.

In countries like France, Spain, Italy, and Greece, the foundations of the Mediterranean Diet as we know it today would be associated with the working or 'poor' classes of society. This is particularly true of France, whose early modern history is defined by class warfare demonstrated in works by authors such as Victor Hugo. While the rich dined on heavy meals of calorie-dense meats and cheeses, the poverty-stricken classes subsisted on vegetables and breads.

Cultural influences have a profound impact on modern diets, most notably on the tiny island of Patellaria, whose diet is influenced by everything from Arabic to Italian cuisine. This tiny island in the Mediterranean was cleared for farming by its people some time around the end of the Bronze Age. Around 860 AD, Arab settlers introduced citrus trees and grapes. By the time of the Napoleonic wars, French cuisine had taken hold. This clash of cultures led to the diet enjoyed by many in the modern era.

It might not surprise you to learn that the diet has garnered some scientific interest. What might surprise you is that the diet has been studied for over 50 years. This interest began in the post-World War II years and has grown in the decades since. Research has shown the Mediterranean Diet decreases the risk of dying from heart disease by 55%, and that it can help lower cholesterol and blood pressure. It doesn't promise 'fast results.' There is no emphasis on a 'magic food' that will rapidly boost your metabolism or 'increase thermogenesis.' Your metabolism works just fine the way it is, and thermogenesis is a byproduct *of* your metabolism rather than a process in and of itself. The only 'key' to the diet is the emphasis on eating well. Later in this book, I'm going to share with you a few recipes that I enjoy regularly, as well as some exercise patterns.

Modern Components Of The Diet

Depending on the version of the Mediterranean Diet you follow, the foods available to you will vary greatly. Despite this, it is generally agreed that there are eight "key components" that form the diet as a whole:

- a high ratio of monounsaturated to saturated fat
- moderate alcohol consumption
- a high intake of legumes
- plenty of grains such as breads and cereals
- plenty of fruit
- plenty of vegetables
- low intake of meats and meat products
- moderate intake of dairy products like milk and cheese

Many modern diet trends encourage you 'cut down on' or 'cut out altogether' one or more food groups. It has even become a trend to ignore food altogether and simply subsist on shakes and pills instead of wholesome food. As you can see from the list of components, the Mediterranean Diet does not cut out or cut down on anything. You do not have to follow a diet plan if you don't want to. If you follow a simple 'this is what I will eat this week' plan, and your dishes follow the above guidelines, your diet is already balanced and healthy. Notice the emphasis on *moderation* in the diet. You do not have to cut out the red wine or beer; you simply have to be mindful of your intake. While studies have shown a little beer or wine every now and again might not be harmful, overdoing it will increase the risk of heart disease and liver problems in the future.

Overall, the Mediterranean Diet has been linked to good health, and I will go into detail about this in the next chapter. In this day and age, good health has gained an association with being young, leaving the older generations out of the equation. While this diet is beneficial for anyone and everyone, I want to show you how it can benefit the men in my age group (50+).

Chapter 2: Benefits

The Mediterranean Diet has a wide range of benefits, which I will cover later in this chapter. For the moment, I think it's important to take a couple of pages to consider nutrition in general. I won't go too deeply into the science, but I will cover a few of the more important vitamins and minerals and how they help the body. The human body needs a variety of minerals and vitamins, also known as micronutrients, to maintain functions such as remineralisation of the teeth. In addition, we also need macronutrients—carbohydrates, protein, and fat. Carbohydrates give us energy, protein helps with muscle and cell repair, and fat helps the body maintain hydration.

Nutrition

There are seven vitamins and minerals considered vital in any diet. While all vitamins and minerals are important to the human body, if your diet is lacking in any of the following seven, you could experience some negative health effects.

- **Vitamin D:** This vitamin plays a vital role in the regulation of calcium and phosphate in the body. It also helps the body absorb calcium. Bones, teeth, and muscles all require vitamin D to remain healthy. A deficiency in vitamin D can cause all kidneys of skeletal problems, such as rickets in children or osteomalacia in adults. Some excellent sources of vitamin D are fatty fish like salmon and trout, egg yolks, and certain fortified breakfast cereals, milks, and juices.

- **Folate:** Folate is a B vitamin often found in the form of folic acid, which plays a vital role in the production of healthy red blood cells. Pregnant women are often prescribed folic acid supplements because it also plays a role in fetal development. However, regardless of age, folate helps in the production of genetic material. Folate deficiency can result in extreme tiredness, pins and needles, and mouth problems. Beans, avocados, dark leafy greens, broccoli, brussels sprouts, and citrus fruits are all great sources of folate.
- **Iron:** Around 70% of the iron in your body is found in the haemoglobin of your red blood cells. Without iron, the body would not be able to produce red blood cells. It also plays a role in immunity, metabolism, brain function, and energy production. A lack of iron in the diet can result in iron deficiency anaemia, which is characterised by chills, tremors, and lethargy. Beans, chickpeas, nuts, red meats, peas, spinach, and dried fruit, along with fortified breakfast cereals, are excellent sources of iron.
- **Zinc:** This is a mineral that tends to be lower in the older population, in particular older men. Zinc is essential because it is found all throughout the body and assists the immune system in fighting off infection, bacteria, and viruses. Vitamin C supplements will typically be fortified with zinc for this reason. Additionally, the body needs zinc to synthesise the proteins necessary in DNA creation. Pumpkin seeds, brown rice, spinach, shellfish, nuts, beans, legumes, green beans, eggs, and tahini are all examples of foods high in zinc.
- **Calcium:** If you have strong bones and healthy teeth, it is likely because you are getting enough calcium in your diet. Most of the calcium in the body is stored in the bones and teeth, supporting their strength and

structure. This mineral works with vitamin D to maintain a healthy skeletal system. Calcium also plays a crucial role in the health of muscles and the nervous system. If you are deficient in calcium, you might experience severe muscle cramps and spasms, a burning sensation in the fingers, and in more extreme cases, seizures. Fortified cereals, broccoli, kale, spinach, milk, yoghurt, cheese, beans, lentils, nuts and nut butters are all great sources of calcium.

- **Magnesium**: This nutrient is essential to bone health and energy production. It also helps calm the nervous system, regulate muscle and nerve function, synthesise protein, and balance blood sugar levels. It is easy to become magnesium deficient because not everyone knows what foods contain it. Some food sources of magnesium include artichokes, spinach, brown rice, almonds, peanuts, cashews, Brazil nuts, and pumpkin.
- **Vitamin B-12:** This vitamin is crucial to making DNA and keeping the nerves and blood cells healthy. There is also some evidence suggesting vitamin B-12 can prevent the onset of osteoporosis, anaemia, and even improve eye health. If you are deficient in B-12, you may experience symptoms similar to anaemia. These include pins and needles, lethargy, and irritability. Poultry, beef, fish, and eggs are all great sources of vitamin B-12.

All of these vitamins and minerals are present and available through the Mediterranean Diet. The diet is rich in protein and vitamin B-12 in the form of eggs and oily fish. You might be concerned about the lack of red meat, which is a primary source of iron. There is limited room for red meat in the diet, but this does not mean you cannot have it. You just need to plan when you want to include it. There are plenty of other sources of iron if you want to completely forgo red meat; for example, chickpeas and red kidney beans are great non-meat sources. Fish does contain a small amount of iron, about 0.3 mg per 100 g, although the current recommended daily allowance is 16-18 mg.

Nutrition for the aging population has become a cause for concern in the last few decades. When I was a kid, I thought I would never get old. Well, here I am, and I'm probably better educated about nutrition and health than I ever was when I was a kid. As we age, our nutritional needs change. We are more active when we are young, and as we get older, we become less active, and our metabolism slows down. We do not need as much energy as we used to. This might suggest that we need to eat less.

However, there have been waves of research into this area. The older body may be less efficient at absorbing nutrients, although nutritional demands may actually *increase*. Everyone has individual nutritional needs based on several factors. Certain age-related conditions require medications that might slow down the metabolism, resulting in weight gain and inefficient nutrient absorption. B vitamins, for example, do not interact well with many medications, so they simply are not absorbed by the body.

This isn't to say that when you get old, your body gives up. There are several ways you can help your body improve metabolic efficiency. Exercise is a great way to get your metabolism moving, no matter your age. There is some evidence that regular exercise can help strengthen the digestive tract. One of the reasons for this is that your blood flow is diverted from the digestive system because the need for it is less urgent.

Nutritional needs tend to differ with gender and age. Some people take it upon themselves to consult a dietician, get blood tests, and tailor their diet as needed. In doing this, they can keep an eye on the levels of nutrients in their blood. While I do not recommend this practice, it *is* helpful to speak with a medical professional and get to know your nutritional needs. Different men need different nutrients, just like an active person might need more calories than a less active person. Take a few hours to examine your lifestyle and try to fit your nutritional needs with your physical needs. If you are quite sedentary, chances are your metabolism isn't that active, which means you won't feel hunger or experience cravings. A more active man who goes to the gym or plays sports on a regular basis will need more protein and carbohydrates because his metabolism is much quicker.

Another nutritional factor people often ignore is keeping an eye on your portion sizes. It's easy to overindulge in a lot of tasty food, and the Mediterranean Diet offers some delicious dishes. It also offers some great opportunities to control your portions. If you go to your local supermarket and pick up, say, a punnet of grapes, you might notice that a 'single serving' is approximately ten grapes. I know a fair few people who will sit and eat the entire punnet over the course of an hour while they're working. Because this diet is so varied in terms of nutrition, you have more options for snacks. Not only this, but the food is much more filling. While protein is not as emphasised as in the keto diet, there is enough to keep you going through the day.

In the next part of this chapter, I want to go over some of the pros and cons of the diet. There are a lot of benefits, the Mediterranean Diet is not without its negatives. While you might enjoy the broad range of food available to you, you might find yourself budgeting quite a bit. That is why I want to cover the negatives, because there are easy solutions to problems that may arise. You have much more to gain from this diet than you might lose.

The Pros

The Mediterranean Diet has a lot of positive things about it. You might have seen it referred to as a diet trend. While it is true that it is quite trendy among the younger crowd, the same cannot be said of the older crowd, particularly middle-aged men. We men tend to be quite simple in what we enjoy, but we enjoy trying new things every now and again. What I've enjoyed most about my own journey on this diet is how much energy it's given me and the variety of food I've been able to enjoy. I started it out of curiosity, and once I noticed how good I was feeling, I wished I had started sooner. The Mediterranean Diet covers all the major food groups: breads and cereals, vegetables and legumes, fruits, dairy, and lean meats and proteins. Not all of these are allowed on other diets. The ketogenic diet, for example, emphasises fat and protein with limited carbohydrates, while the paleo diet stresses 'whole' foods and avoids processed and refined sugars and carbohydrates. Unlike the keto diet, the Mediterranean Diet has more leeway for carbohydrates, where about 50-60% of calories come from breads, vegetables, and fruits. Similar to the paleo diet, one of the core philosophies behind the Mediterranean Diet is about lifestyle changes. Incorporating exercise alongside the diet is pivotal to keeping your body healthy and happy.

Like I mentioned, the diet offers an incredible variety of foods. Unlike with keto and paleo, nothing is off limits, per se. You can even enjoy an optional glass of wine with dinner if you feel like it! Fruits and vegetables get a massive emphasis. Like you were told when you were a kid, you should aim for 'five a day' when it comes to your fruits and vegetables. These are not just a great source of dietary fibre, but also vitamins like vitamin C, vitamin B12, and folate. Not all fruits and vegetables are created equal, however. A carrot contains more vitamin A, vitamin K, and manganese than, say, an orange, which also contains more vitamin C than the carrot. To keep an eye on your portions, always check the back of the package. A 'single serving' will be listed somewhere near the ingredients.

You also have the freedom to enjoy up to three servings of whole grains every day. This could be in the form of some wholemeal, seeded toast with olive oil spread (or butter if you're feeling naughty) in the morning, some brown pasta for lunch, and a side of brown rice with salmon for dinner. Whole grains are probably the easiest to fit into your diet because they are so common. A whole grain is any grain that still contains the endosperm, germ, and bran of the wheat. This is why brown bread and brown pasta are, well, brown. Brown rice is brown because it's a different type of rice. Whole grains contain the unrefined ruffage of wheat, unlike refined grains, which only have the endosperm. There is very little nutritional difference between whole and refined grains in terms of vitamins and minerals, with the exception of B vitamins. The key differences lie in the fibre content, texture, and shelf life. Refine grains have lower fibre, a lighter texture, and a longer shelf life, while whole grains have a higher fibre content, a dense texture, and a shorter shelf life.

Although the Mediterranean Diet has a bit of a bias towards fish and lean proteins, this does not mean you *have* to eat this for every single meal. You might want to follow a plant-based version of diet instead. This might be the case if you're a vegetarian, vegan, or have an allergy to any kind of seafood. Beans and legumes are a cheap, tasty way to get your protein and fibre in one meal. When you hear 'beans,' you probably think of a can of Heinz, which might go on toast or with a Full English. There are actually four hundred kinds of beans, all of which offer different concentrations of vitamins, minerals, and protein. The most popular are rosecoco, chickpeas (also known as garbanzo beans), black beans, kidney beans (which can be red or white), black eyed beans, and broad beans. Because beans and legumes are so inexpensive, you can stock up on them for later use. Beans and legumes are also highly versatile. You can make a meat-free chili con carne with three kinds of beans, replace the lean beef in a cottage pie with some black beans, or have a go at making a lentil dal with some Bombay-style chickpeas. Speaking of chickpeas, you can use the aquafaba from a can of chickpeas (or dried chickpeas, which require soaking overnight) to make some low-calorie, low-fat, high-protein meringues.

In terms of snacks, you don't just have to stick to fruit. Fruit is quite high in natural sugars, which isn't always a good thing. If you want to cut down on sugars, you can always grab a handful of nuts and some seeds. Almonds and Brazil nuts are great sources of natural fats. While they should be enjoyed in moderation, they can be part of a balanced meal. Broadly speaking, nuts are absolute powerhouses of antioxidants. Oxidation is a process in which chemicals change due to the presence or addition of oxygen. Your body needs this to happen, but it can cause a strain on the body and result in the presence of free radicals. This is where antioxidants step in: evidence suggests that the antioxidants present in nuts like walnuts and almonds might help to protect the cells from oxidation. Nuts and seeds are also very filling. If you start to crave sweets, a handful of nuts and a glass of water can help to sway those cravings and keep your stomach satisfied until your next meal.

Fats and oils are another food group covered by the Mediterranean Diet. Although it is not advised to overdo them, the body does need fat to aid in processes such as digestion and hydration. Avocados are a great source of monounsaturated fat, the 'good' fat that helps lower cholesterol. They also contain more potassium than bananas. You can also get avocado oil, which is nutritionally similar to extra virgin olive oil. Extra virgin olive oil is recommended as your primary source of fat while on the Mediterranean Diet, although you are encouraged to explore other types of oils to add some nutritional variety to your meal. In terms of butter and spreads, stick to olive oil spread in place of dairy butter.

Speaking of dairy, while you are allowed dairy products like yoghurt and cheese, enjoy them in moderation. Cheese, for example, has been shown to stimulate the same parts of the brain as hard drugs like cocaine and heroin. A nice piece of cheese on toast is delicious, but because milk is not a traditional part of the Mediterranean Diet, it isn't really recommended. That's not to say you can't enjoy some mozzarella melted over a nice thick piece of brown bread with a drizzle of olive oil. It just means you should keep an eye on your cheese and yoghurt intake. Probiotic yoghurts, for example, are allowed as long as you're aware of your fat intake. If you're struggling to cut out the dairy, try substituting with unsweetened almond or soy milk.

Like dairy, red meat is best enjoyed occasionally. The Mediterranean Diet is based around fresh fruits and vegetables, herbs, nuts, beans, and whole grains, with plenty of sources of healthy fats. Protein is found in the abundance of seafood like fish and shellfish as well as the occasional piece of chicken and even eggs, so the need for red meat is relatively minor. You don't have to give up your Sunday roast, however. A topside of beef or leg of lamb can still be enjoyed in moderation. Studies have linked red meat with heightened risk of death and increased risk of certain cancers, in particular bowel cancer.

Unlike other diets requiring varying degrees of restriction, adhering to the Mediterranean Diet is much easier. Returning to the example of the ketogenic diet, if you were to follow this plan, you would have to limit your intake of carbohydrates so much that it causes your body to start burning fat for energy. Although the keto diet is effective for weight loss, it can result in low blood pressure, kidney stones, and nutrient deficiencies. The body may struggle to burn fat for long periods of time, which is why a ketogenic diet should be done under medical supervision. On the other hand, a Mediterranean-style diet is much broader in terms of what you can eat. There are no real restrictions, just recommended areas where you can cut back or moderate your intake. For this reason, you will find it much easier to stick to the Mediterranean Diet over the long term compared to other, more restrictive diets.

... And A Few Cons

Just like with any diet, there are some downsides to the Mediterranean Diet. They aren't anything serious, just a few things to keep in mind. Before you start any diet, you should always consult a medical professional or dietitian. Get a blood glucose tracker to keep an eye on your blood sugar and get a good MOT from your doctor. A Mediterranean-style diet gets about 35-40% of its calories from fat. While there are documented benefits to heart health, most medical professionals advise keeping fat calories below 35%.

Also keep in mind that this diet can quickly become expensive. In the UK alone, consumer prices for fish have risen dramatically over the decades. This is best reflected in the price of cod. In 1971, the average price for 1 kg of cod was around 53p, compared to 2021 where the price is 1530p (yes, that's £15.30) at the time of writing. Of course, these prices reflect a variety of factors, including running and transport costs. It could also be said that cod is more valuable. Regardless, there are ways you can keep costs down. When you go to your local supermarket, look for 'last day' promotions in most sections. Browse the fish aisle. You might be able to buy some lovely cod fillets for about £3.50 or some fresh salmon for around the same price. Stick them in the freezer the second you get home. Freezing food is a great way to preserve the quality of the fish and keep it fresh. While fresh fish is preferable, it can be cooked from frozen, but this makes it difficult to tell when it's cooked. Fish should be cooked to an internal temperature of 62.8°C (145°F) before it's safe to eat. For this reason, it might be a good idea to invest in a food thermometer.

In terms of vegetables, they've always been pretty inexpensive, but with so many new varieties on the market, it can be difficult to tell. The rise of plant-based or plant-heavy diets has led to an increase in 'vegan-friendly' and 'vegetarian-safe' alternatives for dairy products like yoghurt and milk, causing price increases over the last decade. Conversely, vegetables have remained at a relatively consistent price since 2012. Marketing labels such as 'organic' and 'farm fresh' come with small price spikes. Buy frozen and in bulk if you can. Frozen vegetables like peas and carrots retain their freshness and nutritional value for up to a year after freezing and can be cooked without thawing.

One last thing to consider in terms of expense is supplements. This may or may not be related to the Mediterranean Diet, but taking supplements like iron, vitamin C, and anything you can get over the counter is quite popular. The thing to remember is that the body will always take what it needs from the fuel you give it. However, if you struggle with a medical condition and require supplements, try to get them through an NHS scheme or your health insurance provider. This would be a way to keep supplement costs down, of course. Otherwise, you can shop around for deals on things like orange juice with 'extra vitamin C' or breakfast cereals that have been 'fortified with iron.'

Another drawback of the Mediterranean Diet is the time it takes to cook. Cooking is a wonderful pastime that helps you learn what foods you like and gives you control over your portions. Unfortunately, cooking also takes a good deal of time, which is a luxury some people don't have. A terrific way to make the most of your time is to plan your meals. Take a couple of hours on a Sunday to plan how many onions or cloves of garlic you will need for the week and chop them up, or buy a bag of pre-chopped onions and a jar of pre-chopped garlic in olive oil. You could also plan 'leftover nights,' which are exactly as they sound. Prepare too much on purpose so you can take them with you to work for lunch or have them another night in the week. Most of the recipes I'm going to give you will last three days in the fridge, making them perfect for leftovers.

Returning to the idea of meal planning, you could take a leaf out of the fitness industry's book and actually *prepare* the meals beforehand. Fitness fanatics will use the weekend to prepare all their meals for the upcoming week, but you don't need to do that. You can simply prepare it the day before alongside that day's dinner, or do the prep work for dinner at lunch time, and so on. Also, don't be afraid of freezing your leftovers. Almost everything can be frozen and kept for months before you're ready to eat it again, as long as you don't forget about it! It is true that freezing can compromise the quality of fresh food, but as long as you thaw it out before attempting to reheat it (and make sure that it's heated all the way through!), everything will be absolutely fine and taste terrific.

Something that I want to make clear about the Mediterranean Diet is that it's not designed for weight loss. It's true that you can lose weight while on the diet; this is due to any number of factors. You might notice that you drop quite a few pounds in the first few weeks as your body adjusts and then plateau later. This is normal, but the plateau will continue. The diet is simply designed to be much healthier than a typical Western diet. By tradition and speculation, the typical British diet is very 'meat and two veg.' Potatoes feature quite a lot in the national palate along with red meat like beef and lamb and a lot of poultry and pork. We simply love our meat, but that doesn't mean eating it to excess is good for us. The Mediterranean Diet features something that is sorely lacking in modern British cuisine: variety. Variety in fats, carbohydrates, and proteins, the three big macronutrients the human body needs.

Conclusion

There are many nutritional benefits to the Mediterranean Diet. Due to the variety of foods available, you will generally get everything the body needs to function properly. This is perhaps the greatest benefit of the diet. That, and the diet can be suited to anyone. Of course, seeking medical advice is always a good idea before you start any new diet. You might want to take a blood test and get a general MOT so you can be aware of what you need to include on a daily basis. Dietary needs alter with age, although there are multiple factors at play. Gender, for example. As men get older, the metabolism slows down significantly. This can be corrected through regular exercise, which we will cover in a later chapter. There are several downsides to the Mediterranean Diet, which come down to time and money. However, there are several easily implemented solutions to these issues.

Chapter 3: Recipes

I would like to dedicate this next section to some recipes that I have personally used, as well as a few I am keen to experiment with. You could say that this next section is a bit closer to a cookbook than a diet book. For this reason, I would like to make something clear: the only healthy diet is the one in which you approach food with a healthy attitude. You are *allowed* to enjoy your favourite foods, no matter what the latest fad diet says. That's the reason I included a few sweet recipes at the end of this chapter. While overindulging on cakes and sweets is not healthy, punishing yourself or beating yourself up for every bite you take is even less healthy. Some of these recipes are designed to be healthy in general, like the sea bass recipe. A cooked fillet of sea bass contains 150 calories and can be served with salad and new potatoes. This is obviously a low calorie, nutritious meal. However, the Greek yoghurt parfait recipe might appear unhealthy and full of sugar, but it is full of probiotics from the yoghurt and vitamins, minerals, and dietary fibre from the fruit.

When it comes to food, approach it with the intention that it will fuel your body or give you satisfaction. The phrase 'empty calories' is quite common in the diet industry, meaning something that has a lot of calories but little nutritional value. Cakes are considered to be full of 'empty calories,' but so is olive oil. That's right. Olive oil contains a lot of important fats, but that's it. It's still considered a 'healthy' oil. If you are concerned about your health and are changing your diet to lose weight and become more focused on the nutritional value the Mediterranean Diet has to offer, feel free to skip the pudding recipes. They will still be there if you're ever ready to try them.

Breakfast

Omelette

Eggs make for a great source of protein, but the yolks contain more fat and calories than the whites. A good breakfast or brunch omelette will contain selenium, Vitamins B6 and B12, iron, zinc, and other nutrients. Omelettes are a versatile breakfast food that can be filled with different meats or vegetables depending on your appetite. For a lighter omelette, try adding 2 tablespoons of water, which helps to loosen up the proteins, making them less tough and easier to work with.

Ingredients

- 1 tbsp olive oil
- 3 egg whites
- 2 whole eggs
- ½ tsp garlic sea salt
- 1 handful of spinach
- 1 small onion, chopped
- 4-5 baby plum tomatoes, chopped
- Low-fat grated cheese (to serve)

Method

1. Gently heat the olive oil in a frying pan. While the oil is heating, beat together the egg whites and eggs with the garlic salt until combined.
2. Pour the eggs into the frying pan and allow to heat. Scrape down the sides of the pan and swirl it around to cover the pan. This will help the egg cook quicker.
3. When the egg is cooked most of the way through and still a little runny on top, sprinkle your fillings over one side

of the omelette. Flip the other half over to cover it. Don't worry if the egg breaks—this will resolve itself when you turn it.
4. Let the omelette cook on one side for 1-2 minutes and then flip and cook on the other side for the same length of time.
5. Sprinkle the grated cheese over the top and then flip it one last time to melt the cheese. Decant onto a dish and serve.

Wholemeal Pancakes

The trick to making delicious, moist pancakes is not to overwork the batter. Unlike with cake batter, where you want all of the wet and dry ingredients to get to know each other intimately, overworking pancake batter makes pancakes tough and glutenous. Instead, incorporate the wet ingredients and allow the batter to be a bit lumpy. Let it sit for 10-15 minutes so that the dry ingredients can slowly absorb moisture and then ladle it into the frying pan for fluffy, moist pancakes.

Ingredients

- 128 g (1 cup) wholemeal flour, sifted
- 236 ml (1 cup) unsweetened almond milk
- 1 whole egg
- 2 tbsp sweetener (I use stevia)
- 1 tbsp olive oil
- 1 tsp mixed spice
- 1 tsp sea salt

Method

1. Preheat a frying plan with 1 or 2 tablespoons of olive oil.

2. Pour the flour into a mixing bowl and then slowly add the wet ingredients. Mix together slowly, just enough so that all of the ingredients are incorporated.

Mediterranean Shakshuka

A versatile food, enjoying shakshuka for breakfast sets you up for a good day. Beans offer a great source of protein and are full of dietary fibre. This dish will leave you feeling full and satisfied. Shakshuka has a variety of interpretations depending on the part of the world you are in. If you enjoy a flavoursome curry, substitute the Italian flavours of this recipe with some madras seasoning or the spice palate of your favourite curry! If you want something a little more meaty, cut the beans in half and bulk it up with some chorizo or lean turkey breast.

Ingredients

- 2 tbsp olive oil
- 3 cloves garlic, crushed or chopped
- 1 small red onion, chopped
- 1 can black beans
- 1 can chopped tomatoes
- 1 tsp oregano
- 1 tsp basil
- 2-4 large eggs, depending on the size of your pan
- Sea salt and freshly ground pepper to taste

Method

1. Gently heat the oil in a frying pan and then add the garlic and onion. Sautee them until they go translucent and give off a nice scent.
2. Add the can of beans, fry gently to heat them through, and then add the can of tomatoes.

3. Sprinkle in the seasonings and allow to heat through. Before you add the eggs, make some little holes in the bean and tomato mixture, one for each egg.
4. Crack the eggs into the holes and cover the pan with either a plate or a suitably sized lid, checking every 2-3 minutes. This will poach the eggs and allow them to cook through.
5. Once the eggs are cooked through, remove the pan from the heat and serve with a little optional coriander to garnish. Add salt and pepper to taste.

Oat and Berry Smoothie

This delightful mixture can be enjoyed as either a regular smoothie or prepared the evening before as overnight oats. The balance of carbohydrates from the oats and berries and the protein and fat from the milk and yoghurt offers a nutritious breakfast. You can mix and match the fruits used for this recipe.

Ingredients

- 200 g 0% fat Greek yoghurt
- 250 g frozen berries
- 50 ml unsweetened almond milk
- 2-3 tbsp honey

Method

1. Using an immersion blender, or a regular blender, blend together the berries and milk until well combined.
2. Decant this mixture into a small bowl or a glass, and stir through the oats and honey.
3. Enjoy!

Lunch

Flatbread Pizza

You do not need a takeaway to enjoy a nice pizza for lunch. It's healthier to make your own. Using a premade wholemeal flatbread if you don't feel like making one from scratch is perfectly acceptable, although I prefer making my own. This recipe is high in protein from the chicken and offers a nice balance of fats and carbohydrates. Of course, you are free to customise it as you wish with toppings. Although I recommend olive oil, you might want to try avocado oil or even a nice glug of peanut oil for variety in fats!

Ingredients

- 2-3 tbsp olive oil
- 1 onion, chopped
- 1 wholemeal flour flatbread (store-bought is fine if you don't want to make your own)
- 2-3 tbsp sugar free tomato base
- 1 chicken breast, cooked and shredded
- Handful low-fat mozzarella cheese
- Pinch of rocket, to serve (optional)

Method

1. In a small saucepan, gently heat the olive oil and lightly fry the onion with the shredded chicken breast just for a bit of colour. Spread the tomato base over the flatbread.
2. When the chicken has a nice bit of colour, spread it evenly over the flatbread and drizzle with some olive oil. Sprinkle the low-fat mozzarella over the pizza, covering the chicken.

3. Place under the grill or in an air fryer for 5-10 minutes, or until the edges are nice and crisp.
4. Take it out and serve with a good handful of rocket leaves.

Turkey Burger With Sweet Potato

Turkey is a rich source of protein, niacin, vitamin B-12, vitamin B6, and an amino acid called tryptophan. Enjoying a tasty burger and chips once a week might have been the norm when you were a kid, but now that you're a bit older, it's time to optimise your weekly treat. By making your own burger, you have some control over how the burger tastes and the size of the patty. Serve this with salad or, if you're feeling a bit decadent, a toast wholemeal bun.

Ingredients

- 2-3 tbsp olive oil
- 2-3 large sweet potatoes, chopped (with skin is best)
- 1 onion, chopped
- 450 g lean turkey mince
- 1 tsp mixed herbs
- 2 tbsp wholemeal flour
- Black pepper, to taste
- Sea salt, to taste

Method

1. Toss the sweet potato chunks with some olive oil and a pinch of sea salt, then place in a tray and cook in the air fryer at 280 degrees for 24-30 minutes.
2. While the sweet potato is cooking, take the mince and mix in the chopped onion, sea salt, black pepper, and mixed herbs. Combine until you have a smooth

consistency. Add a couple of tablespoons of wholemeal flour to help bind the mixture.
3. Depending on the size of your patties, this mixture will make up to four small ones or two very big ones. Shape them to your desire.
4. In a frying pan, heat a little olive oil and fry the burgers until they achieve a nice golden colour.
5. Serve with the sweet potato chunks.

Mediterranean Quinoa

Quinoa is a protein-rich grain that has taken the food world by storm. It is wonderfully versatile. Much like arborio rice, its size increases when heated. When cooked according to the package instructions, it can triple in volume. For this reason, you should always cook less than you think you need. This quinoa recipe is ideal for a light lunch, although there are so many components you will feel full! As with any recipe, once you have mastered this basic meal, you can add your own twist to suit your needs.

Ingredients

For the red pepper sauce:

- 450 g roasted red peppers (if using jarred, make sure they are well-drained; otherwise, roast your own)
- 1 clove garlic, crushed
- ½ tsp sea salt, to taste
- Black pepper, to taste
- 1 lemon, juiced
- 7 tbsp olive oil
- 118 g crushed roasted almonds

For the quinoa

- 120 g cooked quinoa

- Good-sized handful of spinach
- 50 g Feta cheese, cubed
- 1 pinch fresh basil or parsley
- 2 tbsp lemon juice, to serve
- 1 tbsp olive oil, to serve

Method

1. In a food processor, pulse the red pepper, oil, garlic, lemon juice, sea salt, and black pepper together until it reaches a thick, lumpy consistency. If you do not own a food processor, mash everything together roughly in a large bowl.
2. Once this has been reached, scoop the cooked quinoa into a bowl and start building around it.
3. Enjoy!

Lemon And Chicken Soup

This is a delicious Greek recipe best suited for the end of winter and the turn of spring. It is full of immunity-strengthening vitamin C from the lemons and muscle-friendly protein from the chicken. If you would like to increase the lemony flavour, go ahead and add some sliced, fresh lemon to the stock and remove them before serving, or serve with a lemon wedge to squeeze over just before you enjoy it.

Ingredients

- 2 tbsp olive oil
- 2 tbsp butter (unsalted)
- 1 onion, chopped
- 2-3 large carrots, chopped
- 1-2 ribs celery, chopped
- 5 cloves garlic, crushed and minced

- 1 tsp ginger, grated
- ½ tsp sea salt
- ½ tbsp lemon zest
- 3 cooked chicken breasts, shredded
- 1 litre low-sodium chicken stock (homemade or store-bought is fine)
- 1 low-sodium stock cube (like OXO or Knorr)
- 500 ml water
- 70 g orzo
- Fresh herbs, chopped (basil, parsley, thyme)
- 3 tbsp grated parmesan cheese, to serve

Method

1. In a large pot, gently heat the olive oil and butter together. When the butter is melted, add the onion, carrots, celery, garlic, ginger, and salt and pepper. Cook for about five minutes or until the vegetables are slightly soft. Stir frequently to avoid burning.
2. Add the lemon zest and chicken and cook until the chicken has a nice light brown colour. Pour in the stock and water, along with the low-sodium stock cube. Bring to a boil.
3. Once the mixture is boiling, add the orzo and reduce the heat to simmer. Cook for 8-10 minutes, or until the pasta is al dente. At this stage, add the herbs and chives. Top with the parmesan cheese and serve immediately.

Dinner

Tuna Pasta

A simple recipe, the staple of many British dinners, tuna pasta offers both nostalgia and nutrition. Tuna is packed full of omega-3 fatty acids, and the wholemeal pasta will increase your fibre intake. This is a basic recipe that you can customise to your personal tastes. You can substitute the tune for tinned salmon, for example. If you would like to add some vegetables, a chopped rib of celery and some tinned sweetcorn will provide some texture as well as taste.

Ingredients

- 250 g dried wholemeal pasta, any shape
- Salt, to taste
- 1 tin tuna in brine
- Sea salt, to taste
- Black pepper, to taste
- Handful of rocket leaves, to serve

Method

1. Cook the pasta according to package instructions. Add a pinch of salt to the water if desired.
2. Drain the cooked pasta and allow to cool. Drain the brine from the tuna and mix it into the pasta along with the sea salt and black pepper.
3. Serve with a handful of rocket leaves to garnish.

Pan-fried Sea Bass

While this one is not a complete meal, sea bass is an excellent source of potassium, selenium, protein, and magnesium. A fatty fish, you will also get a good dose of omega-3 fatty acids.

You can get fillets or whole sea bass at your local supermarket from anywhere between £3.70 to £10, depending on the species and quality. The amount you spend doesn't matter; you will still get the same nutrition. Pan-fried sea bass goes well with wilted spinach and fresh red onion, some citrus-dressed broccoli, or a nice refreshing salad.

Ingredients

- Sea salt
- 2 fillets fresh sea bass (frozen and thawed is also fine)
- 2 tbsp olive oil
- 1 lemon, cut into 8 wedges

Method

1. Heat up a frying pan until it is very hot. While it is heating up, season the sea bass fillets with the sea salt.
2. Add the oil to the pan then place the fillets skin-side down. To stop it from curling up, gently press the fillets down with your fingers. If you are not confident using your fingers, use a fish slice.
3. Reduce the heat to medium and allow the fish to continue cooking until you can see that ⅔ of the flesh is cooked. This should take about 4-5 minutes.
4. Flip the fillets over to the flesh side and allow to continue cooking for 2 minutes. Remove from the pan and allow to rest on a warm plate. To keep it moist, baste with the oil and juices from the pan. I recommend using a pastry brush to do this.

Baked Lemon And Garlic Salmon

Salmon is a popular fish, and it might just be the most nutritious fish you can eat! Rich in everything from protein to

B vitamins to omega-3 fatty acids, adding salmon to your diet two or three times a week will help support your overall health. This recipe is simple and can be made either in bulk or individually. I encourage you to experiment with the flavour profile of this dish. Lemon and garlic are such a classic combination for salmon, but experimenting with other types of citrus will unlock entirely new experiences. A nice pungent horseradish marinade will add a bit of kick, but those who feel like being a bit sweet might want to experiment with a little drizzle of honey.

Ingredients

- 2-3 tbsp olive oil
- ½ tsp black pepper
- 1 tsp paprika
- 1 tsp oregano
- Pinch of sea salt
- 4 cloves garlic
- Juice of 1 lemon
- Zest of 1 lemon
- 1-4 salmon fillets (one per serving)

Method

1. Preheat the oven to Gas Mark 5 and prepare a baking tray with a large piece of foil (or baking paper if you have it).
2. In a small bowl, make the sauce. Combine the lemon juice, paprika, garlic, and oregano.
3. Depending on the number of servings you want to make, take the salmon fillet(s) and drizzle with a little olive oil. Brush down the baking tray with some olive oil as well and then rest the salmon on top of it. Either brush the sauce over the salmon or pour it over in a nice, even coat.

4. At this point, you can add some optional slices of lemon. Salmon is quite delicious on its own, but you can't over-lemon it! Wrap the foil over as though the salmon is a small package.
5. Bake the salmon at Gas Mark 5 (375 degrees if you are using an air fryer) for 15 minutes. If your salmon is thicker than 1.5 inches, cook for a little longer.
6. Remove from the oven and place under the broiler or exposed in the air fryer for a couple of minutes so that it develops a nice colour. Serve with some orzo salad or seasonal vegetables.

Roasted Mediterranean Vegetables

These crisp vegetables can be enjoyed as part of a larger meal or on their own. Roasting is a cooking process, ideal for slow cooking. When vegetables are roasted, their natural sugars are released. Although all vegetables contain water or some type of moisture, this cooks off quickly, and the caramelisation of natural sugar creates that lovely golden brown colouring. You can most clearly see this transformation on root vegetables such as potatoes, although onions also caramelise very easily. This effect is less pronounced on mushrooms, which are mostly water. This recipe is versatile, so you can use any combination of vegetables.

Ingredients

- 1 small butternut squash, cubed
- 1 large red onion, cubed
- 150 g mushrooms, whole or cut into quarters (your choice!)
- 1 courgette, cut into 1-inch slices
- 2 red peppers, chopped into large pieces
- 4 tbsp olive oil

- 4 cloves garlic, crushed and roughly chopped
- 1 tsp oregano
- 1 tbsp basil
- 1 sprig fresh thyme, chopped
- Sea salt and black pepper to taste

Method

1. Preheat the oven. In a large bowl, mix the oil with the garlic, basil, oregano, sea salt, and black pepper.
2. Put your vegetables into the bowl and toss until they are well-coated with the oil mixture.
3. Spread them out evenly on a baking tray. Sprinkle over the thyme and then roast at Gas Mark 5 for 30-45 minutes, or until slightly charred at the edges. If using an air fryer, roast at 300 degrees for 20 minutes or until the hard vegetables have some give when pierced with a knife.
4. Take them out of the oven and let them cool. Enjoy as a side or on their own!

Orzo Salad

Orzo is a funny little pasta shape. You would be forgiven if you mistook it for rice because the shape is so similar. In fact, 'orzo' is the Italian word for 'barley,' so the pasta shape actually resembles barley grains. It's not suited for something like a Bolognese, but it's perfect for seasonal salads. Salads do not have to be lettuce and tomato. Adding orzo gives a great sense of texture, and a squeeze of lemon juice will add a nice bite, complimenting the spinach. This salad offers a variety of nutrients from the combination of veggies and some healthy fats from the olive oil. For some extra healthy fats and a fresh taste, serve with half an avocado.

Ingredients

- 25 g dry orzo
- 10-12 cherry tomatoes, halved
- ½ can chickpeas, drained and rinsed
- 1 small cucumber, peeled and chopped
- 1 tbsp basil, fresh and chopped
- 1 small red onion, chopped
- 28 g baby spinach (optional)
- 2-3 tbsp olive oil
- Juice of half a lemon

Method

1. Cook the orzo. Do this by placing it in a pot and covering it with water. Allow it to boil, then reduce the heat and simmer for 8-9 minutes or until tender. Drain the orzo and rinse with cold water.
2. In a large bowl, combine the orzo with the tomatoes, (optional) spinach, chickpeas, cucumber, basil, and red onion. Toss them together.
3. Drizzle in the olive oil and toss again, then add the lemon juice and toss one last time before serving.

Sweets And Puddings

Olive Oil Brownies (makes 16 brownies)

Brownies are a decadent treat with a fudgy centre. By replacing the butter in the recipe with olive oil, you can cut down on the amount of fat you are eating. While this does not necessarily make them healthier (remember, there is still a lot of sugar and chocolate to consider), the olive oil makes them more moist. Brownies made with butter dry out after a couple of days in storage, but oil is more stable and helps the brownies maintain their fudgy texture. Light olive oil has a subtle flavour, so it doesn't offset the chocolate.

Ingredients

- 120 ml light olive oil
- 2 tsp vanilla extract or flavouring
- 150 g caster sugar (substitute with your preferred sweetener)
- 90 g brown sugar
- 3 large eggs
- 40 g cocoa powder
- 70 g wholemeal flour
- 75 g chocolate chips (optional)

Method

1. Preheat the oven to Gas Mark 4. If you are using an air fryer, skip this step as you will be baking the brownies at 180°C. Prepare an 8-inch baking pan by lining it with baking parchment.
2. In a large mixing bowl, combine the olive oil with the vanilla, caster sugar (or sweetener, if using), and brown sugar. Mix them together for a couple of minutes.
3. Crack the eggs into a separate bowl and beat them for 30-45 seconds with a fork or until they are a pale yellow colour.
4. Pour the eggs into the large bowl, along with the cocoa powder, wholemeal flour, and chocolate chips if you are using them. Gently combine the mixture using a silicone spatula.

5. Decant into the baking pan and bake for 27-30 minutes, or until a knife inserted into the middle comes away clean. Allow the brownies to cool before removing them from the pan. Slice and serve with either cream or ice cream, or enjoy on their own.

Greek Yoghurt Parfait

This simple pudding could also double as a breakfast. While dairy intake is limited in the Mediterranean Diet, you can still enjoy it in moderation. Greek yoghurt offers some great probiotic properties, while the fruit provides some texture to the dish. You can enjoy this as a pudding in the summer or as a breakfast. This recipe is ideal for one person as a breakfast or two people as a pudding.

Ingredients

- 1 banana, sliced
- 50 g fresh raspberries
- 50 g fresh strawberries, hulled and cut into quarters
- 100 g 0% fat Greek yoghurt
- 1 tbsp honey, to serve

Method

1. In a bowl, scoop in about ½ of the Greek yoghurt. Add a small layer of banana slices, some of the raspberries, and the strawberries.
2. Add the rest of the yoghurt and top with the remaining fruit.
3. Drizzle the honey over the fruit and serve.

Italian-style Vanilla Cheesecake

Most cheesecakes use cream cheese, but using ricotta makes for a creamier, more subtle pudding. Known for its subtle taste, ricotta can be used in a variety of sweet and savoury dishes. Ricotta also contains less fat than cream cheese. If you want to keep an eye on your fat intake or want to cut back on calories, use a low-fat, low-calorie ricotta.

Ingredients

- 100 g granulated sugar (or your preferred sweetener)
- 45 g all purpose flour
- 450 g ricotta
- 2 tsp vanilla extract
- 5 eggs
- 2 tsp citrus zest (any, optional)

Method

1. Preheat your oven to Gas Mark 2 and prepare a springform pan. Brush down the sides with a little oil and lining with some baking paper, cut to size.
2. In a large mixing bowl, gently combine the flour and sugar using either a whisk or a fork. Add the ricotta and vanilla, as well as your optional zest, and combine.
3. One at a time, add the eggs, stirring between additions. Pour the cheesecake into the pan and bake for 80-90 minutes, or until the top begins to turn brown.
4. Check that the centre of the cheesecake is firm enough by sliding a knife into it. If the knife comes out clean, it's ready. Let the cheesecake cool on a wire rack, then cover and refrigerate until you are ready to serve. You may notice that it shrinks a little as it cools. This is normal.

Blood Orange Olive Oil Cake

Blood oranges contain a great deal of vitamin C, vitamin A, and dietary fibre. Of course, this cake also contains a fair few calories per slice (around 230). This is a decadent cake best enjoyed with friends and strong coffee.

Ingredients

- 300 g caster sugar (or your preferred sweetener)
- 5 large eggs
- Zest and juice of 3 blood oranges
- 150 ml olive oil (preferably light)
- 280 g self-rising flour

Method

1. Preheat your oven to Gas Mark 4 and prepare a cake tin. Brush it down with either a bit of olive oil, or spray it with a cake-release spray. You could also use baking paper.
2. In a mixing bowl, beat together the eggs, zest, and sugar with an electric whisk until thick and pale. Pour in the juice and oil and mix until well combined.
3. Sift in the flour and mix until a smooth batter is formed.
4. Pour the mixture into the tin and bake for 40 minutes, or until a utensil inserted into the centre comes out clean.
5. Allow the cake to cool before slicing and serving.

Snacks

A lot of foods fall into the 'snack food' category when it comes to the Mediterranean Diet. However, you are advised to avoid processed foods. Instead of a bag of crisps, which are full of unhealthy oils and loaded with sugars and sodium, you can have a go at baking your own potato crisps with a sprinkle of olive oil and sea salt. Potatoes are allowed on the Mediterranean Diet because the diet has a lot of room for healthy starchy vegetables, and as a versatile root the potato can be turned into all sorts of tasty treats. Thick-cut chips fried in a little olive oil and baked, for example, can still be enjoyed with a nice fillet of salmon.

For a slightly healthier fix, you can enjoy a handful of baby carrots with some hummus. Hummus does contain a lot of fat from the oil it uses as a base, so try to find a low-fast option to enjoy. In addition to the baby carrots, toast up some wholemeal flatbread or a pita and cut it into thick strips. If you would like to avoid the crisps, as with the first example, this is an acceptable substitute. Not only is it crunchy, but you cut out the artificial flavourings and gain the fibre from the bread and vitamin A from the baby carrots. Celery and broccoli stems, which you can slice up into thin strips, make great snacking veggies. Regarding broccoli, you might be like most people who don't know what to do with the stems once you've trimmed off the florets. The stems can be eaten raw or fried in olive oil and enjoyed as a side. It's edible and delicious!

Nuts and seeds are packed with vitamins and minerals. Toasted pumpkin seeds are a great source of calcium—100 g of them contains about 20 mg! Nuts, in particular Brazil nuts, almonds, and peanuts, are also high in naturally occurring fats and sugars, so you should moderate your intake of them. Almonds are probably the best nuts to snack on, and almond butter makes a great substitute for peanut butter if you are trying to cut back on sugar in general. Some sliced green apple with almond butter is a great snack in the spring.

Even though you are eating a healthy diet, you should never forget to stay hydrated! Avoid drinks that contain added sugars.

While you can enjoy fruit juice, go for a reduced sugar option or a sugar-free squash. Although you are allowed up to one glass of red wine per day, you should aim to avoid this if you have a history of alcoholism or are trying to avoid alcohol in general. Perhaps the most important thing is to drink plenty of water and keep a chilled water bottle with you at all times.

Conclusion

You can enjoy a variety of meals on this diet. It doesn't have to be all fish and vegetables with a bit of fruit every now and again. Low-fat Greek yoghurt is a healthy alternative to heavy cream in a lot of dishes. Quinoa provides a protein boost. Beans are cheap and plentiful in variety. Fish and poultry can be bought for cheap if you know where to look. The emphasis on whole foods and fresh vegetables and fruits is what makes this diet so nutrient-dense. Of course, this can have a few unpleasant side effects to consider, which we will cover in the next chapter.

Chapter 4: Things To Expect When You Change Diets

When a fitness enthusiast starts the ketogenic diet, they experience a collection of symptoms that appear a few days after they begin the diet. These symptoms include headache, fatigue, irritability, nausea, foggy brain, insomnia, and constipation. Collectively, these symptoms are referred to as 'keto flu.' However, this is not a medically recognised condition. These symptoms occur because the body no longer has carbohydrates to burn. Instead, it has to burn ketone bodies. One of the reasons behind this is that there are temporary imbalances in energy and mineral levels in the body and disturbances in hormone balances. For example, insulin production is disrupted because carbohydrates are needed for the process.

Changing your diet is going to cause all kinds of changes to the body. Depending on where you are in the UK, the average British diet is full of refined carbohydrates and saturated fats. According to the latest data, this could explain why more than 60% of Britons are overweight or obese. Of course, factors such as physical activity and lifestyle choices also affect this. This notwithstanding, poor diet is the leading cause of a variety of health problems in the UK. A poor diet can cause heart disease and diabetes, both of which are on the rise in certain parts of the country. A recent study suggests that while most 19-64 years olds are getting more than their 'five a day' in fruit and vegetables, the groups in the 65+ range are struggling to meet their dietary requirements.

Although the national diet has improved over the last few years, according to the National Diet and Nutrition Surveys conducted between 2018-2020, consumption of sugary drinks and high-fat foods is still something of a problem among certain demographics. Britons love their processed meats like sausages, bacon, and mincemeat. We also love baked beans, starchy potatoes, pies, a good pint, and lots of tea. This might look like the diet you currently enjoy. However, it is not healthy. When you switch from this sort of diet to one high in nutritional value, plenty of dietary fibre, and lots of oil fish, your body is going to react to it. The body has its own detox systems, so don't think you need to buy special teas and coffees to 'flush out' your system. I can tell you from personal experience, and plenty of evidence to back it up, that these substances only cause you harm. They work by causing excessive urination and diarrhoea. You lose water weight and, when you stop taking the tea, you will just gain it all back, just like with yo-yo dieting.

Something you might notice when you first start eating healthily is you will feel hungry. Rest assured that this is normal. More specifically, you will start to crave the foods you are cutting back on. The Mediterranean Diet focuses on whole grains and whole foods in general, so when you go from eating refined carbohydrates like white pasta and white bread, and switching them with brown pasta and brown bread, your body will notice. White bread causes a prominent and immediate sugar spike in the body, while brown bread takes longer to digest and is more sustained over the course of the day. Your body will miss the immediate sugar spike, causing you to crave high-sugar foods and drinks. When this happens, increase your water intake. Drink a few sips of water with lemon juice for flavour. Additionally, the lemon juice will help settle your stomach.

A second, slightly more embarrassing, side effect of switching to the Mediterranean Diet, is that you will experience bloating and flatulence. Again, this is completely normal. Your body is experiencing an influx of dietary fibre from fruits and vegetables, in addition to lots of fish, which is quite soft. All of this will result in some slight disruptions to your digestive system. The addition of a probiotic yoghurt, as well as watching your portions, will help to improve the flatulence. Bloating occurs when intestinal gas and food block up the lower intestine. Again, this is happening because of all the fibre you are taking in. Drink plenty of water, get a bit of light exercise in, and it will resolve in a few days. Another approach you could try, if you have a bit more patience, is to implement your new diet slowly. Instead of switching overnight, gradually incorporate more fruits and vegetables into your diet, slowly remove certain dairy products, have fish once a week instead of every night. It can be tempting to just rush in, but when you do this, you will end up with bloating and flatulence. If you do, try to stay away from social gatherings for a couple of weeks while your body adjusts!

You might also notice changes in your mood. It is not true that you only use 10% of your brain at any one time. In fact, your brain is constantly working. Picture your car, if you have one, or anything that has an engine. To keep running, that engine requires fuel, and that fuel needs to be of good quality in order for the engine to run efficiently. The same is true of your brain. You may have heard of dopamine, the 'reward' chemical. Dopamine makes us feel good and encourages us to repeat specific behaviours in order to stimulate its release. Serotonin is a neurotransmitter, 95% of which is produced in the gastrointestinal tract. From this information, we can guess that the food we eat can also help guide our emotions. When we eat refined carbohydrates, the brain releases dopamine because it recognises that there are lots of calories and a quick source of energy within this food. As a result, we are encouraged to repeat the behaviour. When we remove refined carbohydrates from our diet, the body almost goes into shock because it is trying to find the refined carbohydrates it's used to. Because it can't find them, we don't get the dopamine drop. Depression or low mood can result from this. If you feel depressed, consult a medical professional immediately.

You might also notice that you lose weight quite quickly at the start of a new diet. While this is unconfirmed in the case of the Mediterranean Diet, rest assured that this is also normal. You could lose up to two kilograms (just under 5lbs) in the first week. However, do not expect this to continue. The weight you are losing is water weight. This occurs when the body starts dipping into its stores of energy, known as glycogen. Glycogen is bound to the water molecules in your body, so when the body burns the glycogen, it also releases the water. You might experience frequent urination as a result. This is just another way you might shed the water weight. As your body adjusts to its new diet and the new sources of energy available to it, your weight will plateau, and you will start to shed the pounds at a regular, steady rate.

After about 21 days, your body will have adjusted to a healthier diet. Since the Mediterranean Diet contains more nutritionally valuable foods than the average British diet, you can expect that the above symptoms will last for around a month. Research suggests that it can take up to 18 weeks to break a bad habit such as eating unhealthy food or cutting back on sugar. There is also evidence to suggest that, at least in the case of switching diets, gradual change is more sustainable than an overnight 'cold turkey'-style shock to the system. At around the four-week mark, your body will start to absorb more nutrients, and you will feel healthier. Your mind will feel less foggy, your energy levels will increase, and your metabolism will start to pick up. The Mediterranean Diet is full of nutritious food, so do not be surprised when the benefits all come at once.

And that's about all you can expect when you change diets. It's tempting to make the change to a healthy diet immediately, but the fact is the human body is not equipped for overnight changes. It's built for periods of fasting and to burn energy efficiently, but making a sudden dietary change can cause a lot of digestive problems. While you will experience changes to your mood, it is important that you seek medical attention if it gets too rough. Drink lots of water, get plenty of exercise, and be patient. Good things will come!

Chapter 5: Intermittent Fasting

The practice of fasting is not new. It has been a part of human history for millennia. Hippocrates, after whom the Hippocratic Oath is named, prescribed fasting as a medical treatment. Other philosophers followed his lead. Plato said, 'I fast for greater physical and mental efficiency.' There have been several studies into how fasting can be used to assist with mental health and neurological diseases. Something that has been well-documented is the improvements made to 'cognition, age-related cognitive decline, slowing of neurodegeneration, reduction of brain damage, and the enhancement of physical recovery after a stroke.' The study these results were taken from was performed just a couple of years ago, in 2019. This study, and several others, have noted a sharp increase in the production of brain-derived neurotrophic factor (BDNF). This is a protein which, in humans, promotes nerve growth, neuroplasticity, and cell maturation. It also plays a complex but vital role in cellular repair.

Taking in massive amounts of food regularly results in a myriad of health complications. This does not mean that you should restrict your calories. Extreme calorie restriction, the opposite end of extreme calorie intake, results in similar health complications and other, more serious problems. Eating too much increases the risk of developing heart disease, obesity, and diabetes. Eating too little leads to muscular atrophy, cardiovascular problems, and oxidative damage. Intermittent fasting offers a healthy middle ground between eating and resting. By fasting, we are helping the brain keep itself in shape. The production of BDNF allows the brain to increase the resistance of its neurons. In 2018, Mattson *et al* identified that the most affected processes are mediated by the central nervous system. This sort of activity has been linked to increased neural functionality. In simple terms, it helps your brain work better. It should be noted that a majority of the studies were performed on animal models. At the time of writing this, research is ongoing into the effects of fasting in human models.

Intermittent fasting is an eating pattern and a common sense one, at that. There are different 'patterns' to it. When I say 'patterns,' I really mean that there are several popular ways to implement intermittent fasting into your daily routine. Depending on the model you choose, you might have an easier time than you think. Or, you might have a difficult time. Practice makes perfect, as they say. Some models require keeping a reminder on your phone or a note on your fridge to keep you on track, while others are a bit more 'common sense.' When you start any new eating regime, you should always consult your GP or a dietitian. You should do this especially if you are on medications that need to be taken with food. Once you've had your consultation, you can pick a method which is suitable for you, or you can give each of them a go for a few weeks and see which is best suited to your lifestyle.

There are actually six very popular methods.

16:8

The most popular method of intermittent fasting, the 16:8 method is a daily fasting/eating schedule. It involves a 16-hour fasting window and an 8-hour eating window. There are plenty of ways to implement this pattern. For some, it could be as simple as skipping breakfast and deciding to say 'no' to seconds or pudding after dinner. You might find this method difficult to implement if you enjoy eating a big meal for breakfast. If this applies to you, enjoying a fruit and oat smoothie or a low-calorie protein shake in place of a large meal is a useful 'cheat.' However, this might be a great option for you if you don't enjoy eating in the morning. Some ways to subvert feelings of hunger (which you *are* going to feel, especially if you're normally a breakfast eater) include black coffee, herbal teas, black tea, lots of water, and zero-calorie drinks. Most people put their fasting window in the night to coincide with when they're asleep.

5:2

This one is one of the more controversial fasting patterns. It involves eating normally five days a week and having two days where your calorie intake is restricted to 400-600 calories. You can choose which two days you lower your calorie intake. You might eat a normal diet every day except for Mondays and Thursdays, for example, when you would eat low-calorie versions of your favourite foods or subsist on low-calorie snacks. I hope it's obvious why this is a bit of a controversial method of fasting. There are currently no studies that examine the effectiveness of the 5:2 pattern. While it has been shown that a calorie deficit does support weight loss, there is no evidence to support that a 'normal' diet with two integrated low-calorie days is any more beneficial.

Eat Stop Eat

This fasting pattern was popularised by a prominent figure in the fitness industry, and it may be the most challenging. It involves a 24-hour fast from 7 p.m. to 7 p.m. So, from dinnertime to dinnertime. A popular fasting window for this one is also breakfast to breakfast. Since you will not be taking any solid food, it is recommended that coffee, zero-calorie drinks, and plenty of water continue to be a part of your routine. Unlike the 16:8 pattern, there is little evidence suggesting any long term health benefits. Although it does encourage a calorie deficit and places the metabolism under mild stress, resulting in a faster calorie burn rate, all of the evidence is circumstantial or anecdotal.

Alternate Day Fasting

Fasting every other day can seem like it's a bit extreme, although different variants of this pattern exist. Some might allow up to 1000 calories per day. Others might have a 'smoothies only' option. Trepanowski *et al*, and other studies examine the effects of alternate day fasting over short periods of time. As yet, there are no long-term studies. Trepanowski *et al* discovered that a zero-calorie fast on fasting days was more likely to fail due to the high demands being placed on the body. At the same time, the two calorie-restriction groups were able to maintain their schedule and lost similar amounts of weight. If you decide to try this variant of intermittent fasting, set yourself a calorie limit and use a calorie tracker.

Warrior

This variant of intermittent fasting became popular only a few years ago. The fasting/eating pattern is 20:4, so a 20-hour fasting window and a 4-hour eating window. It involves eating only small amounts of fruits and vegetables with some dairy products in the fasting window (typically from breakfast to an hour before dinner) and a large meal at dinner time. There is some evidence demonstrating short-term weight loss and maintenance of blood glucose, but there is no evidence to support weight loss in the long term; nor are we certain about the long-term health effects.

Spontaneous Skipping

Some people enjoy having a structure to their fasting, while others need the degree of flexibility offered by spontaneous skipping. This one might actually be the better option for anyone who skips breakfast. The human body is well-equipped to deal with famine, but skipping too many meals can result in the body going into starvation mode. Under spontaneous skipping, if you've eaten a lot during the day and don't feel like eating dinner, you can skip it. If you're taking a long train journey from King's Cross to Edinburgh and don't fancy anything in the concessions carriage, you can do a short fast. The flexibility offered by spontaneous skipping is useful if you have a busy life.

What To Expect When You Start Intermittent Fasting

Depending on your current level of health, physical activity, and the nutrition in your diet, you might not experience any side effects. You might experience a little extra hunger in the evening as you go to bed or the morning as you wake up. This is because your body is getting used to a new pattern of nutritional intake. Breaking habits like having a few cheese and crackers before bed because 'the cheese helps me sleep' sends the body into a state of alarm because it was expecting that intake of fat. Intermittent fasting on the 16:8 pattern could help you break this habit.

If you are currently not physically active or your overall diet is quite poor and a bit all over the place, intermittent fasting can help you establish a routine. You may experience some side effects such as extreme hunger pangs and resultant mood swings as your body adjusts to its new way of processing food. Common side effects also include feeling mentally and physically sluggish. Research suggests that it can take the body two to four weeks to adjust to intermittent fasting. This is not a 'lose weight fast' solution; it's a pattern of eating. When you start any diet regime, you will always experience a huge drop in weight loss at the very start. After this, you will hit a plateau of 0.5-1kg per week. This does not mean that intermittent fasting or your diet has stopped working. It just means your body is used to its new way of eating. It's a good thing!

Metabolism is the series of chemical processes by which the body converts food into energy. A simple example is the conversion of glucose into glycogen, which is then absorbed into the muscles to power the cells. Part of this involves the fed-fast cycle. There are four stages: feeding, pre-absorptive, fasting, and starvation. During the feeding state, the body is receiving nutrition. Then it moves into the pre-absorptive state, where digestion prepares the nutrients in food for absorption into the body. Fasting typically occurs at night when we sleep. Humans almost never enter the starvation stage of the fed-fast cycle, as this is where the metabolism starts to 'eat itself.' Intermittent fasting focuses on cycling the first three stages of the fed-fast cycle as it keeps the metabolism at a sustainable work:rest ratio.

Stockman *et al* (2018) reviewed a variety of intermittent fasting patterns, including the variants I listed above. The findings were mixed, and Stockman *et al* conclude that further research is needed due to the small or moderate sample sizes and short duration of each study. What they also found was that, depending on the model of intermittent fasting, the benefit-to-harm ratio also varied and was affected by factors including genetics, age, gender, and environment. Women over the age of 40 tend to do better with the 16:8 pattern, while men have more success with spontaneous skipping, depending on the study you read.

The Benefits Of Intermittent Fasting

The main reason people swap to intermittent fasting is for weight loss. While weight loss is an evidence-backed side effect of this eating pattern, it's not the only one. Losing weight often happens at the start, and it's more noticeable for that reason. As I mentioned before, you start to hit a plateau with the weight loss aspect of intermittent fasting. Once this happens, you begin to notice the *other* effects it has on your health.

Just to warm us up, I'm going to remain along the thought of weight loss for a second and talk about muscle mass. When bodybuilders are 'bulking up' for a show, they increase their protein intake and cut out all of the good stuff. Protein is great for building muscle, but what it also does on a body builder's diet is provide a calorie surplus. If you need a calorie deficit to lose weight, you need a calorie surplus to gain weight. This is what's meant by 'gains' in the fitness industry. Your body uses a lot of energy when healing all of the microabrasions in the muscle fibres, which is why so many calories are needed. Assuming you're active, you probably have a decent amount of muscle mass that you don't want to lose.

Numerous studies have examined the influence of diet and lifestyle changes on weight loss and muscle mass. One such study by Varady *et all* (2011) took two groups of people, all of whom were obese, and put them each on the same 12-week exercise programme, but gave one group an intermittent fasting schedule while the others had more freedom. The study discovered that both regimes helped each group lose weight, but the key difference was in muscle mass. The group who had more freedom over their dietary habits lost both body fat *and* muscle mass, while the group who fasted did not lose muscle mass, just the fat. For that reason, if you're looking to trim up for a summer trip to Brighton Beach, intermittent fasting is an effective way to maintain your muscle mass.

This next change is on a much smaller scale, quite literally! While you might not be able to see the changes, you will certainly feel them. Intermittent fasting has been shown to have a significant effect on the way our hormones work. Most notably, insulin. Insulin is the hormone that helps your body maintain its blood sugar levels. Alirezaei *et* studied the effect of intermittent fasting in mice back in 2016. Mice have similar biological mechanisms to humans, which gives researchers a good idea of how changes like intermittent fasting *might* be applied to humans. This study showed that blood insulin levels dropped dramatically, suggesting stability in blood sugar levels. With Type 2 diabetes on the rise in the UK, it has become increasingly important for men over 50 to keep an eye on their blood sugar levels. One of the dangers of diabetes, in general, is the risk of insulin resistance. When this happens, the body simply stops responding to insulin, which means that the cells can't get the energy they need to function. Alirezaei *et al*'s study was just one of many that identified the effectiveness of fasting on blood sugar levels. This also means that you are at less risk of developing Type 2 diabetes in the future. Differences between men and women are still being investigated, with strong evidence that blood sugar control is more prominent in men.

When you hear about 'inflammation', you probably think of it as something to avoid. Inflammatory foods such as gluten and certain spices can cause gut problems and the like. However, inflammation is not always detrimental. It's the body's natural response to infection, illness, and even injury! If you sprain your ankle walking down the stairs, it becomes *inflamed* because you've sustained an injury. When you get a cold or the flu, your chest and lungs become *inflamed* as they work to fight off the sickness. If you've ever had a nasty cut that turned red and swollen, and you had to be prescribed antibiotics to fight off infection, it was *inflamed*. Inflammation is natural, but that doesn't mean it's entirely good. Arthritis is a painful disease that causes moderate to severe inflammation in the joints. Chronic inflammation occurs when the body is fully healed, but the inflammatory response remains. Because of this, the body stays on high alert, prepared for the next infection or injury. Both arthritis and chronic inflammation are painful, stressful illnesses that can be made worse by common household foods like table sugar (glucose), trans fats, and refined carbohydrates, all commonly found in a Western diet heavy in fried, fatty, and sugary foods.

One of the other side effects you are bound to notice is an improvement in your inflammatory response. Arthritis typically develops in older individuals, particularly men over 50, although younger people can develop it too. Several studies have found that inflammation of this nature can be reduced by intermittent fasting. This works by reducing overall oxidative stress, which is the relationship between free radicals and antioxidants in your body. To put it simply, free radicals can cause damage to your cells, while antioxidants help with cellular repair. Oxidative stress is a leading cause of inflammation, and intermittent fasting can help improve the body's resistance toward it.

I think that these are among the best side effects of intermittent fasting. They aren't immediately obvious, but after a few months, you will start to notice the changes occurring in your body. Along with the exercises, which I will get to in the next chapter, this will help improve your overall health.

Conclusion

There are plenty of benefits to intermittent fasting, including improved blood sugar regulation and weight management. Although the practice of fasting is not new, the way we use it to benefit our health is. Most of the methods I have shown you are quite common sense. For example, fasting at night and not eating until a little while after you've eaten. Some of them require a lot of patience to implement, while others are less demanding. If you are new to intermittent fasting, I recommend doing the 16:8 pattern. However, I do not recommend taking it on at the exact same time as starting the Mediterranean Diet. Start it a few weeks before so your body can adjust to your new eating pattern. As you start to implement healthier foods, you will begin feeling lighter, healthier, and more energetic.

Chapter 6: Get Moving!

If you're anything like me, the last time you *properly* exercised was your very last PE class, and the thought of exercise now fills you with a sense of dread. One of the things you'll notice while on the Mediterranean Diet is that you will regain your energy. You won't be buzzing like when you were younger, but it will be a nice stable sort of energy that encourages you to push a little bit more. The better fed your body is, the better it will move. All of the omega-3 fatty acids in your diet will start to help your joints feel a bit smoother, and the influx of B vitamins will help you feel a bit more awake. For this next chapter, I want to take you through some exercise options. There are plenty of free workouts available on YouTube, many of which are hosted by well-known UK gyms such as PureGym and the Gym Group.

You may have an emotional block, or maybe you're recovering from an injury that makes it difficult to move. You could also team up with a friend if you aren't confident enough to start on your own.

Some Great Ways To Move

When you start working out, you have to make sure that you are doing what's right for *your* body. If you want something that focuses on muscle building, resistance training might be the way to go. For fat burning, you need to give cardio some thought. Whatever your goals, there is an exercise to accommodate it. I find that alternating between different types of exercises encourages the brain and body to work together, maximising the benefits from each.

Yoga

Yoga has a variety of health benefits, from reducing body-wide inflammation to improved cardiovascular health. Practicing yoga on a regular basis acts as a form of body conditioning. Depending on the type of yoga, the benefits can change. Ashtanga yoga, for example, is quite intense and relies on consistent movement. You typically hold a downward-facing dog for a few breaths before moving on to a new pose. Conversely, Yin yoga is much slower and allows you to relax into the pose before moving onto the next one. A Yin flow is focused on a slow, steady pace that challenges the mind as well as the body.

Practicing yoga is particularly good for men in their 50s because it improves your flexibility and strength. You might associate yoga with the younger crowd and their expensive coffee and avocado toast, but they *are* onto something with yoga. If you go onto YouTube, you can find various flows that focus on different body areas. Hip-focused poses such as 'Lotus' or 'Happy Baby' stretch the hip flexors and strengthen the surrounding muscles as well as the pelvic floor. After a flow, you will notice that you stand up straighter. This is because many positions strengthen core and back muscles. With a stronger core, you end up with a much healthier posture.

Part of the body's natural stress response is to release cortisol, high levels of which can have negative effects on the body. Regular yoga practice has been linked to reduced levels of cortisol. One study evaluated such effects on a group of people on a six week yoga retreat. Some of the participants practiced once a week, others practiced one flow every day of the study, and the rest practiced every other day. By the end of the six week retreat, the groups who practiced yoga more often had less cortisol in their system than the participants who practiced once a week. By incorporating yoga into your exercise routine, you can improve your stress levels. This will translate into improved heart health because cortisol is one of the hormones responsible for tightening arteries during cardiac arrest.

HIIT

High-Intensity Interval Training (HIIT) is a style of exercise that focuses on fatiguing the body in a short period of time. There are various styles. For example, cardio HIIT will focus on calisthenics and anything that gets the heart racing and the blood pumping. Other types of HIIT workouts include resistance training. HIIT has some incredible benefits. If you are looking to increase your health and athleticism, HIIT is the way to go. Studies have shown that it can increase your VO2 max, which is your maximum oxygen consumption during exercise. As the name implies, all exercises must be performed at high intensity. While this sounds intimidating, it's far more achievable than you might imagine.

Let's say you're doing a routine that includes star jumps. On your first round, you might manage 12 star jumps in 30 seconds. The goal for the next round would be to push that to 13, then 14 on the next round, and so on in that fashion. HIIT has become a longstanding workout trend which has gripped plenty of fitness fanatics, old and young. This is due in no small part to the fact that it encourages you to push yourself. While you won't see results from it for the first two to three weeks, you will notice the internal changes. Since your body is getting so much more oxygen, your brain will start to function more efficiently. On a cellular level, your metabolism will be more effective. Combined with the benefits of intermittent fasting, you stand a much greater chance of fine tuning your body.

The goal of HIIT is to burn fat and build muscle—fast—and you don't need to spend hours in the gym to do it. You can do it just as easily at home in 20-45 minutes. Bear in mind that with each round, you *have* to increase the level of intensity. If you are doing HIIT with weights, this could mean performing reps at a faster speed, or it could mean adding an extra weight plate with every round. When doing cardio, you might start off at 60% effort, but you *have* to end at 100%. Remember, the goal is to become *fatigued* by the end of the session. If you have access to a gym, check out their class schedule and attend a few of their HIIT classes to get an idea. This will help you build your own workouts later on. Or if you don't feel like going to the gym, you can check out YouTube or download an app.

Weight Training

Training with heavy weights or any kind of resistance has its origins in Ancient Greece, where the Olympics originated. Although they would not have used anything like a barbell or a gym standard weight plate, the Ancient Greeks made ingenious use of what we would consider everyday items. For example, it was not uncommon for an Olympic wrestler like Plato to train his power by throwing a weighted bag of sand from one side of the room to another. In place of dumbbells, the Greeks lifted heavy stones known as *halteres* to target their biceps and triceps. Ancient Olympians trained with weights for their specific sports. And now, millennia later, the ancient Greeks might be agog to see how many options we have for weight training. We have weight machines where you can load up plates, barbells that can be adjusted, dumbbells of varying weights, medicine balls, resistance bands, and even weights to suit your ankles and hands for an added bit of resistance. These tools are not only available in gyms; you can invest in yourself and get some good quality weights for a reasonable price—if you have space in your home, of course. A barbell, for example, measures around seven feet long depending on the type of bar. Olympic barbells and hexagonal barbells are popular models and offer different benefits depending on the exercise being performed. Many exercises, such as a shoulder press or pectoral fly, can be performed with a set of dumbbells.

Weight training is not only good for the muscles; it's good for the body overall. Any form of exercise will help reduce blood sugar levels, but weight training has been shown to help people maintain a strong level of stasis. Weight lifting also burns significantly more calories than cardio. Cardio is great to get your heart pumping, but weight training will continue to burn calories for hours after the workout is done. Continuing with the metabolism, your body has a basal metabolic rate which burns between 1800-2500 calories depending on a variety of factors including, but not limited to: gender, lifestyle, level of activity, diet, and present environment. When you do cardio, you can burn a lot of calories very quickly, and your basal metabolic rate increases for a few hours afterwards. When you do weight lifting, however, your basal metabolic rate peaks and continues to run at a heightened level for up to 48 hours.

The important thing about weight training is that you keep pushing yourself. When your body gets used to a certain amount of weight or a specific routine, it might feel good for the brain, but the body has already optimised itself for that specific sequence of events. To put it simply, it stops working hard. You might mistake this as a sign that your body is getting stronger, when actually it's getting a bit lazy. When you take up weight lifting, you might get into the habit of doing, say, three sets of 15 Romanian deadlifts and four sets of 15 back squats at 15kg. This is a great place to start! However, if you want to push yourself, you need to do one of three things: increase the weight, increase the reps, or increase the intensity.

Adding extra weight plates to your bar might seem like an insurmountable challenge, when actually it's just giving your body a little something extra to push against. If you feel discomfort at any time, it is okay to set down the weight or adjust the weight you're lifting. The saying, "no pain no gain" has some truth to it, in that if you're sore the next day it means you did something right. However, if you're in pain *while* exercising, it's time to stop, grab some water, and catch your breath.

Cycling And Spinning

Whether you have an old bike you haven't used in years, or you want to invest in one of those fancy new stationary bikes with the TV screen attached to it, cycling and spinning are a couple of great exercises. Although they primarily work the lower body and leg muscles, cycling and spinning have a range of cardiorespiratory benefits. The difference between these two exercises is that cycling is a bit more high impact since you are dealing with going up and down hills, while you can control the resistance with a stationary bike, making it lower impact.

Another benefit of cycling and spinning is how good they are for the joints, particularly the hips. Since it doesn't overstress the leg muscles, you can expect to experience more mobility in your hips and knees for days after a session of spinning or cycling. While cycling or spinning will not give you super powerful legs, you can maximise the benefits by adding in a few squats, donkey kicks, and lunges.

You can do either cycling or spinning as part of a team. Joining a local cycling club is a great way to meet new people and make friends, while spin classes tend to have a lively vibe where the instructor encourages you. Some will even walk around the class and adjust your posture as necessary. In addition, spin classes tend to be done in a high-intensity interval format, which not only helps you burn fat but increases your endurance. This can apply quite well if you choose to go for a bike ride around your local park or down a country road.

Swimming

If you want a full-body experience as you exercise, swimming is a great, medium-intensity, low-impact way to get moving. You do not need to be an expert to swim, but if you are feeling less than confident in your ability, look for swimming lessons in your area. It may have been a while since you last had a swimming lesson, and trust me it's easy to forget what you're doing when you hit the water. Swimming can be such a good exercise that within a few months, you can experience a great transformation.

Swimming helps to keep your heart rate up while also taking a lot of stress off the body. You mainly use your arm and leg muscles to keep moving, although you are forced to use your core in order to stay afloat. As a result, you build up your endurance and muscle strength, as well as your overall fitness. You do not need to swim every day to feel the benefits; once or twice a week will do when done as part of a varied regimen.

Most swimming pools will offer water aerobics classes for older people. These exercises are low impact, and the added resistance of the water helps to improve your balance, coordination, muscle strength, and it is much easier on the joints in general. Another benefit of these classes is that they get you out of the house, so you can get your warm-up in with a short walk if it's near where you live, or a nice bike ride if you have a bicycle.

Bodyweight Exercise

You do not need to go to the gym and break out the barbells and dumbbells to get a good workout. Working out at home can be just as beneficial. Bodyweight exercises are simply exercises done without any form of resistance. Actions like pull ups, push ups, squats, situps, and lunges can all be done without adding resistance. The weight of your body provides all the resistance you need.

Working out with nothing but your bodyweight offers a lot of benefits. Most notably, these exercises encourage you to work *with* your current weight rather than *against* it, so the effects adapt to your body. This develops your muscle strength and cardiovascular fitness all in one go. You might also notice that most high-intensity interval classes focus on bodyweight exercises. This is because it's easier to transition between exercises while also getting the heart racing.

The best benefit of bodyweight exercise is that it's free if you do it at home. Countless personal trainers have uploaded exercise videos to YouTube and other video-sharing platforms. You can follow along on these or find exercise plans online.

Alternatively, if you can afford it, you can hire a personal trainer and ask them to focus on bodyweight exercises.

Cardio

Regular cardiovascular exercise is important. Not only is it great for lowering blood pressure and strengthening the heart, but also it is a terrific way to get the metabolism moving. Although we will cover running, a popular cardio exercise, there are more types of cardiovascular exercise that you can and should explore. Most high-intensity interval training regimes you find online will include several heavy cardiovascular elements, such as star jumps, side skaters, or mountain climbers, which are said to 'amplify' the bodyweight portion of the exercise. Medical experts advise at least two hours of moderate aerobic, or cardiovascular, exercise a week. This could be in the form of running, cycling, swimming, or even playing football with your friends.

One great benefit of cardio exercise is that it can help improve the quality of your sleep. A 2010 study by Reid *et al* investigated the effects of regular moderate cardio on individuals with chronic sleep issues. The participants were split into two groups: one group performed regular moderate cardio exercise, and the others were a control group. The study lasted 16 weeks. Overall, the group who performed regular cardio exercise reported that the quality of their sleep improved and extended in duration. Exercise in any form results in the release of energy. For this reason, you should avoid exercising too close to bedtime. Allow your body a four-hour 'cool down' period between exercise and sleep.

Aerobic exercise has also been shown to assist with weight regulation. If you want to focus on calorie burning and endurance building, stick to weight training. A 2021 study by Donnelly *et al* asked overweight participants to maintain their daily diet while engaging in exercise sessions five times a week for a duration of 10 months. At the end of the study, the participants showed significant weight loss, on average between 2-3kg (4-6lbs) compared to their starting weights. The exercises in question encouraged burning between 400-600 calories per day. Further research shows that a calorie deficit in addition to aerobic exercise significantly improves the chances of losing weight and keeping it off.

While exercise in general has been linked to improved mood, cardio has perhaps the highest success rate. One study by Dimeo *et al*, participants who suffered from depression were asked to walk on treadmills while doing intervals for 30 minutes per session. They were asked, after 10 days had passed, to report changes in their mood. All participants reported that they experienced a significant reduction in their depression symptoms. While this is just one study, these results do suggest that engaging in any sort of exercise can have a significant impact on mood. It is generally accepted that it takes up to two weeks to see any sort of improvement to health, whether it's physical or mental. That said, this study also showed that your mental health might improve after a single session.

One reason for this might be the improvements in brain function. A study that investigates this theory involved older participants. While there was no exercise involved, they were submitted for MRI (magnetic resonance imaging) scans. The study revealed that the adults who were the most physically fit, engaging in the most exercise, had fewer reductions in the frontal, parietal, and temporal areas of the brain. This might not sound that impressive, but you should remember that around the age of 50, the grey and white matter of the brain begins to deteriorate. Whatever the reason, aerobic exercise is good for the brain.

So what are some effective, readily available cardio exercises to try out? Swimming is a great, all-round exercise that offers some great aerobic benefits. Going for a 30-minute swim two or three times a week offers similar benefits to high-intensity interval training. If you are not confident with your ability as a swimmer, I advise signing up for lessons, or finding a water aerobics class nearby. Additionally, you might want to try spinning or cycling. Good-quality stationary bikes, which you would use for a spin class, can cost between £150-300, depending on where you get it. Downloading an app or finding a spin class on YouTube is a great way to start! Many stationary bikes have magnetic resistance knobs that increase or decrease the resistance, mimicking the feeling of going up or down hills. Alternatively, you could get some fresh air by investing in a bicycle. The two exercises offer the same benefits.

Running

Going for a light run a couple of times a week is a great way to keep your heart rate up, burn some calories, and see more of your local area. If you have any rivers or natural trails nearby, go for a run along them! Running is a great way to relieve stress on both your mind and body. Like with weightlifting, you can apply some high-intensity intervals while running. You might want to run at a slow, even pace for about half a mile before having 45 seconds to a minute of running at maximum speed.

Running offers a wide variety of benefits. To name one, it strengthens the core and lower body. In 2018, Ponzio *et al* cross-examined 625 marathon runners with the same number of non-active control participants. The purpose of this cross-examination was to determine the flexibility and overall health of the participants' knees and hips. What Ponzio *et al* discovered was that marathon runners had healthier knees and hips than the non-active controls. There may have been other factors related to this, such as diet and training. A diet rich in omega-3 fatty acids, such as the Mediterranean Diet, has also been linked to healthy joints. When you go running while enjoying this diet, you are adding years of life and strength to your knees.

Keeping with the theme of strength, running tones your calves like you would not believe. Ancient marathon runners, who relayed messages from Athens to the city of Marathon, and Olympic sprinters are depicted in ancient art as having powerful legs but flimsy upper bodies. The leg muscles—the quadriceps, hamstrings, and glutes—are responsible for supporting your body while running. Since your legs are moving so much, they have to work extremely hard. The more you run, the stronger they get.

However, it is important to note that there *is* such a thing as too much exercise. At most, you should run three times a week, not just with running but with any exercise. This will give your body a chance to cool down and relax. Stretching is also important. Lactic acid, a byproduct of anaerobic respiration, builds up in the muscles and can cause damage, resulting in cramps and side stitches. Yoga is not only a great way to strengthen and tone the muscles; restorative yoga and hatha yoga are both smooth and easy, focusing on stretching the body and removing tension. If you don't feel like doing yoga, focus on stretching out the calf muscles and the quads, then do a few gentle hip rotations to release the hip flexors.

Just some general advice, on a hot summer day or early spring, when hay fever season is starting to kick in, wear a cloth mask to protect yourself from pollen and pollution. You might feel a bit silly doing it, but this is a trick used by modern day-Olympic athletes! Sporting goods companies have a wide range of filtered masks which are best suited to endurance sports like running.

Elevation training masks, or altitude masks, are designed to simulate high-altitude conditions to increase the stress on your body. This can include lowering the oxygen intake, which forces your lungs and heart to work much harder. Wearing a mask like this purely to make the exercise harder seems counterproductive, but flexibility is about more than just the muscles and tendons. This is not dissimilar to an oxygen hunger exercise. In an oxygen hunger exercise, you might hold a pose (like in yoga), exhale until your lungs are completely empty, and then hold your breath for a count of five. The result is quite painful because your body and your mind are fighting. Wearing an elevation training mask is not quite as painful because you are still inhaling. You're just getting less oxygen than you would normally. Elevation training masks are primarily used by professional athletes or people who are training to climb mountains, but casual fitness enthusiasts have taken an interest in them recently.

Walking

Walking is a great, low impact alternative to running. It's a lovely pastime, especially when the weather is lovely and warm. If you want to control your weight. Walking for around 30 minutes a day a few times a week can help you burn about 150-200 calories, depending on your pace. A slower, more leisurely pace along the river will burn more than a rampant speed walk through the local shopping centre, for example.

As society has progressed and our options for entertainment have increased, many of us have settled into a sedentary lifestyle, especially after age 50. Walking is a great way to break this monotony. Walking is much more relaxing than running and can still improve the overall health of your heart and lungs, which can translate into a lessened risk of heart disease, stroke, and hypertension. You might not immediately feel the benefits of walking, but you will feel your heart rate start to pick up.

Another benefit of walking is the improvement of joint and muscle health. Muscle stiffness, for example, occurs after extended periods of inactivity or after lifting weight that is too heavy. While rest and stretching will help with recovery, walking will help much more. This is because walking for a short time will slowly stretch the muscles and stimulate blood flow. Like with yoga, you might also notice an improvement in your balance.

One benefit of walking, which is true of most forms of cardiovascular exercise, is that it can help improve your immunity, particularly with regard to a cold or the flu. A 2011 study by Neiman *et al* tracked 1002 participants. The group was a mix of men and women and spanned a variety of age groups. Some of them walked at a moderate pace for 20-45 minutes per day, while others either had free reign over their exercise or remained sedentary for the duration of the study. Overall, the group who walked were less likely to get sick with the flu or other kinds of respiratory infections. Additionally, any symptoms they *did* experience if they got sick were far less severe compared to the sedentary group. Flu season is nobody's favourite, and it always happens when the weather is at its worst! This doesn't inspire the desire to walk outside, so you can try walking on a treadmill at the gym or a cheap home treadmill. If you feel like going for a wander somewhere that isn't home, a shopping centre can be a great place to go for a walk.

As I've already mentioned, walking can offer many of the same benefits as running; it's just lower impact. Yoga can be high impact depending on the flow you're doing, while running places more stress on the joints and carries the risk of muscular strain. Ultimately, if your goal is to lose weight, you are better off running a couple of times a week because the benefits are effectively doubled. However, you might be completely new to all forms of exercise or in a position where you are unable to run, so a walk is a great place to begin.

General Activity

It's a common misconception that you have to burn a crazy number of calories at the gym, go running every day, and nearly break yourself lifting heavy weights in order to get fit and lose weight. While this can be the case if you have specific goals in mind, this is not necessarily the case. Even as you're reading this book, your body is burning calories. It's called your basal metabolic rate, and it's the rate at which your body burns calories when you are not moving. Burning calories when performing exercise like high-intensity interval training, weightlifting, or even doing yoga, can help put you into a calorie deficit and even help you burn fat. However, it's not the only way to improve your basal metabolic rate.

All you need to do to keep your basal metabolic rate is simply *keep moving*. I remember years ago, cereal boxes used to have 'healthy guidelines' printed on the back for kids to read, and they would include things like, 'do your homework', 'play some sports,' and 'do the housework.' I can't say if this is still the case, but those old cereal boxes do have a point, and it's backed by scientific evidence. Just keeping active, no matter what you're doing, can improve your overall health. Let's say you're doing the gardening, just pulling up some weeds and getting the soil ready to plant some roses for the next season. You're burning calories and exerting a pull force on the weeds, working your arm muscles, and getting some fresh air at the same time!

Physical activity in any form is great for your health. It does not have to be hardcore, and it does not have to make you sweat buckets. The average person can burn up to 300 calories just by doing the housework. Although housework can be quite sweaty, depending on a number of factors, including the season and how much effort you're putting in, you're still moving and burning calories. You are also making your living environment much healthier by decluttering, using antibacterial cleaning spray, and removing excess dust.

A Note On Safety

As we age, our bodies naturally get weaker. Although exercise like walking and running can help strengthen the muscles and improve athleticism, if you haven't exercised in a long time (or ever!) you shouldn't try to go too hard too soon. There are lots of reasons why you might not have exercised: lack of time, recovering from an intense procedure, not enough energy, to name a few. You might want to run the London Marathon at some point in the future. Best of luck! But you can't expect to immediately run 26.2 miles (42 kilometers) after sitting on the couch for 20 years. Start by going for a slow jog, no longer than 2-3 miles at a time. Build up your endurance and slowly start working in some interval and distance drills. If you need to, see the input of a personal trainer.

Of course, that's just the example of a marathon. What happens if you want to be an older weightlifter? We've all seen the feel-good images and news stories of people who started weightlifting in their 40s and entered their first competition in their 60s. Again, that's a great goal to strive for, and I wish you the best of luck, but you can't load an Olympic bar with 200 kg and expect to lift it on your first day. Weightlifters train in a variety of ways, although they do have to push themselves a lot in order to beat their personal bests. Just remember to start slow.

Yoga is probably the only form of exercise you can practice safely from the start. That said, you need to keep an eye on certain positions. When you're in pigeon pose, for example, you're working your hip flexors and the quadriceps. You should feel a slight stretch in the muscles, just enough that it feels uncomfortable but not painful, but if you feel anything straining or like it's about to rip, move out of the pigeon and straight into the child's pose, a recovery pose. There are a lot of free flows and routines available online. If you need support, try to find a class nearby or hire a yoga instructor who specialises in older clients.

When you start exercising after being sedentary or doing minimal activity, it's tempting to jump right in. The risk of injury is at its highest when you take this approach to exercise. Going too fast on the treadmill can cause a lot of damage to the lungs; lifting too heavy can tear your muscles or strain your back. There are so many things that can go wrong. We spend most of our lives sitting, whether that's at work or at home or out with friends. Sitting is the most common sedentary 'activity' among adults. Although this might feel like a new thing, this has actually been studied since the later half of the 20th century! The results since then have been rather consistent, showing that sitting for extended periods of time doubles the risk of cardiovascular disease. Being physically active is a great way to cut your risk of cardiovascular disease, but it is also a shock to the system.

Getting ready to be active after a long period of going without requires a lot of willpower. All of those young people on social media post pictures of their perfect day where they're doing yoga at the crack of dawn or just finishing their 12th marathon. While some of those posts are fake, the fact that they have the dedication to keep going out and doing it is something to admire. There *is* something to learn here: choosing to exercise is just that. A choice. And you owe it to yourself to be safe. Stretch before you exercise, warm up your joints, start your run slowly. Take a few minutes to check in with your body and mind any injuries.

After a workout, your muscles are going to ache, your lungs will feel raw, and you will be in dire need of a good shower. For any aches and sprains, take a bag of frozen vegetables or an ice pack and place it over any part of your body that feels painful. Extensor tendonitis, which occurs when your tendons become inflamed, is a common injury. It can happen when your shoes are too tight or when you're overworking your legs. The solution for this is to apply an ice pack and keep your foot elevated. If your shoulders are hurting, apply a heating pad.

Another thing to look out for is light-headedness. This happens when you overexert yourself and is common in group exercise classes. Trying to keep up with everyone instead of going at your own pace is probably the worst thing you can do when you first start exercising as it raises your blood pressure. When this happens, lie down in the recovery position and take deep, even breaths. Take some water when you feel better, and seek medical attention if it persists.

Finally, on the topic of medical attention, make sure to get an MOT with your GP before you start exercising. This way, you can get an idea of your current health and fitness level. If possible, speak with a dietitian and a personal trainer so you can get an idea of what sort of exercise will most benefit you. Cardio is the first thing people think of when they want to lose weight and get fit, and while it is a great way to zone out, it's not for everyone.

Conclusion

One of the benefits of the Mediterranean Diet you will experience is an increase in energy. This is due to the influx of nutrients your body is receiving. To amplify the effects of the diet, it's recommended that you take a regular amount of exercise. All exercise offers great benefits, some more than others. It all depends on the goals you have set yourself. You might want to become more flexible or develop your relationship with your body, for instance. This is a goal which can be met by doing half an hour of yoga every day, or an hour three times a week. Plenty of free yoga classes exist on YouTube and various apps you can download onto your phone or tablet. Alternatively, if you want to build your strength, weight training is your best option. Investing in some good quality weights and loading up an exercise video is a great way to get your body engaged. Remember to warm up and cool down, and to not overdo it. Weight training comes with its own set of risks, such as pulled muscles, strains, and (in more extreme cases) breaks. If you want to work in some cardio, walking and running offer similar benefits. Walking is low impact and offers all of the same benefits as running. However, running will help you burn twice as many calories if this is your goal.

Seeking medical attention and considering your current physical condition are both crucial steps to take before you start to exercise, particularly if you aren't used to moving. The sedentary lifestyle is common largely due to the nature of most office jobs, the rise in television as a form of entertainment, and general lack of energy. Jumping straight into marathon training or attempting to get ready for a weightlifting competition too soon can cause a significant amount of damage, so it's important to speak with medical and fitness professionals about your goals before you begin.

Setting goals is an important part of exercise. It's not as simple as getting on the treadmill and just running until you're as buff as Arnold Schwarzenegger. Building muscles takes a lot of time and energy, developing your cardiac health takes patience, and building your flexibility takes months (or even years) of dedicated practice. Before you start exercising, take a few days to consider your goals and plan around them. And, as always, remember to stretch. This will release the lactic acid that builds up in your system and will prevent injury.

I know a lot of people dread exercise, the older generation probably more than anyone. You don't have to go to the gym or go running three times a week. The important thing is to keep active. Whether you're gardening, doing your housework, a bit of DIY on a lazy Sunday, taking the stairs instead of the lift, lifting up the sofa to get your dog's favourite toy, it doesn't matter. As long as you are moving, you are exercising. Eating well can help you maintain your weight or, if it's your goal, keep you in a calorie deficit. Having enough sleep will also help significantly. Remember, if you're in a calorie deficit to lose weight or reduce fat, make sure that it's a gradual process.

Reduce your calories slowly until you've hit your goal. To maintain muscle, gradually increase your protein intake.

Conclusion

The Mediterranean Diet is a name for the way nations along the Mediterranean coast eat. It's nothing special, just a more common-sense way of eating than we might think. With its emphasis on fresh vegetables, whole grains, and oily fish, it might seem too simple to be effective. However, just because it seems simple doesn't mean it can't be varied. I included a chapter dedicated to recipes precisely to show you how varied this diet can be. You do not need to spend an excessive amount on fish every week to enjoy it, and you don't need to have a farm in your back garden to enjoy fresh vegetables on a regular basis. The diet also allows tea and coffee in moderate amounts.

Following this diet has a wide range of benefits. It can assist with lowering your cholesterol, maintaining your blood sugar levels, and dropping some weight. While all diets can be well-balanced, this is probably the only diet that is nutritionally complete without any major adjustments. Several of the major vitamins and minerals are found in foods available within the diet. Oily fish is rich in omega-3 fatty acids. Whole grain breads and pastas are full of dietary fibre and carbohydrates. Of course, if needed, you can take supplements as directed by a medical professional.

Intermittent fasting is simply a schedule for eating and not eating. While there is limited evidence to suggest that it can help you lose weight, there is data that strongly suggests it can help you maintain your weight and even improve your blood sugar levels. There are many ways to implement intermittent fasting, the most popular being the 16:8 split, which means eating a healthy diet for eight hours and abstaining from food for 16 hours (including while you sleep). If you choose to do this, make sure to stop eating an hour before you go to bed and allow your body to 'wake up' a bit before you start eating.

Your nutritional needs change as you get older; that's just a fact of life. As we get less active, our muscles begin to atrophy, we need less iron, and we generally just lose our appetite. This is partially due to the slowing of the metabolism, the sum of all chemical reactions in the body that result in energy production. Regular physical activity can help to improve the metabolism, giving you more energy and better overall health.

There are some negatives to the Mediterranean Diet, but they are easily managed. Preparing your meals ahead of time, whether it's the meal in its entirety or just chopping some vegetables in advance, shaves off a lot of cooking time. Budgeting is also your best friend when it comes to the diet. Good quality fish can be expensive, and the prices will only continue to rise. Shopping in the 'last day' section of your local supermarket is great for both your brain and wallet. Keep any 'last day' cuts of fish in your freezer and make sure they are fully thawed before cooking them.

When it comes to exercising and movement after being sedentary for an extended period of time, for any reason, your safety is key. To avoid muscle injuries, stretch before and after working out. You do not need to spend an arm and a leg on monthly gym fees in order to exercise, unless your goals require you to go to the gym. Going for a walk can give you all the same cardiovascular benefits as a run, for example, and you can get some affordable weightlifting sets online if you want to build up a home gym. Yoga is a great exercise for flexibility, and there are several flows online that target the older generations.

I wrote this book for men in my own age group, the over 50s, because we tend to be forgotten when it comes to healthy living, eating, and exercise. Even if you are living a healthy lifestyle, it could always be healthier. I know from personal experience that some 'healthy' diets are actually unhealthy in more ways than one, particularly for the bank account. This might also be your experience. Or you could be a retired athlete wanting to keep your health in check. Again, see a medical professional if you are concerned about anything. Although a healthy diet plays a vital role in your overall health, it is not the only factor. Exercise also helps, but again, unless you have an idea of what your body needs and is capable of, it's not much use to change your diet and immediately hit the gym. The best form of weight loss and health improvement is slow, gradual change. Your results may not show immediately, but they will eventually build up and start to show.

I shouldn't have to remind you that this is not a miracle diet. It is a matter of making a few lifestyle changes and continuing to eat in a healthy way while getting in some good exercise. As your body adjusts to this new way of eating, you *will* lose *some* weight in the first few weeks, but this will start to even out after a month or so. Do not be disheartened! Health is more than just the number on a scale or the size of your jeans. This is why speaking with medical professionals is so important. Getting a regular check-up to monitor your blood pressure, glucose levels, and cholesterol will give you a better idea of your overall health than stepping on a scale ever will.

Best of luck!

References

Batacan, R. B., Duncan, M. J., Dalbo, V. J., Tucker, P. S., & Fenning, A. S. (2016). Effects of high-intensity interval training on cardiometabolic health: a systematic review and meta-analysis of intervention studies. *British Journal of Sports Medicine, 51*(6), 494–503. https://doi.org/10.1136/bjsports-2015-095841

Best Italian Orzo Salad. (2020, January 24). Creme de La Crumb. https://www.lecremedelacrumb.com/best-italian-orzo-salad/

Blood orange & olive oil bundt cake. (n.d.). BBC Good Food. Retrieved April 30, 2021, from https://www.bbcgoodfood.com/recipes/blood-orange-olive-oil-bunt-cake

Burn Calories With Household Chores. (n.d.). WebMD. Retrieved April 30, 2021, from https://www.webmd.com/fitness-exercise/ss/slideshow-calories-burned-by-household-chores

Calories Burned Cleaning | Calculator & Formula. (n.d.). Captain Calculator. Retrieved April 30, 2021, from https://captaincalculator.com/health/calorie/cleaning/

Casas, R., Sacanella, E., & Estruch, R. (2014). The Immune Protective Effect of the Mediterranean Diet against Chronic Low-grade Inflammatory Diseases. *Endocrine, Metabolic & Immune Disorders-Drug Targets, 14*(4), 245–254. https://doi.org/10.2174/1871530314666140922153350

Chertoff, J. (2018, September 24). *Which Is Better for Your Health: Walking or Running?* Healthline; Healthline

Media. https://www.healthline.com/health/walking-vs-running

Curb, J. D., Wergowske, G., Dobbs, J. C., Abbott, R. D., & Huang, B. (2000). Serum Lipid Effects of a High–Monounsaturated Fat Diet Based on Macadamia Nuts. *Archives of Internal Medicine, 160*(8), 1154. https://doi.org/10.1001/archinte.160.8.1154

Everything to know about The Warrior Diet. (2020, December 22). *Medical News Today.* https://www.medicalnewstoday.com/articles/warrior-diet

Gore, M. (2019, April 29). *This Turkey Burger Is Killer*. Delish. https://www.delish.com/uk/cooking/recipes/a30193110/best-turkey-burger-recipe/

Gunnars, K. (2020a, January 2). *6 Popular Ways to Do Intermittent Fasting.* Healthline. https://www.healthline.com/nutrition/6-ways-to-do-intermittent-fasting#TOC_TITLE_HDR_6

Gunnars, K. (2020b, April 20). *Intermittent Fasting 101 — The Ultimate Beginner's Guide.* Healthline. https://www.healthline.com/nutrition/intermittent-fasting-guide

Harvard Health Publishing. (2015, July 16). *Nutrition and Aging - Harvard Health*. Harvard Health; Harvard Health. https://www.health.harvard.edu/aging/nutrition-and-aging

Harvard Health Publishing. (2018, November 7). *Foods that fight inflammation - Harvard Health*. Harvard Health; Harvard Health. https://www.health.harvard.edu/staying-healthy/foods-that-fight-inflammation

High intensity interval training (HIIT): Benefits and how to start. (2020, January 13). Www.medicalnewstoday.com. https://www.medicalnewstoday.com/articles/327474

Hiraoka-Yamamoto, J., Ikeda, K., Negishi, H., Mori, M., Hirose, A., Sawada, S., Onobayashi, Y., Kitamori, K., Kitano, S., Tashiro, M., Miki, T., & Yamori, Y. (2004). Serum lipid effects of a monounsaturated (palmitoleic) fatty acid-rich diet based on macadamia nuts in healthy, young Japanese women. *Clinical and Experimental Pharmacology & Physiology, 31 Suppl 2*, S37-38. https://doi.org/10.1111/j.1440-1681.2004.04121.x

Homemade Flatbread Pizza Recipe. (2020, April 1). Sally's Baking Addiction. https://sallysbakingaddiction.com/homemade-flatbread-pizza-recipe/

https://www.facebook.com/verywell. (2019). *Should You Try the Warrior Diet?* Verywell Fit. https://www.verywellfit.com/the-warrior-diet-4684768

Institute of Medicine (US) Food Forum. (2010). *Nutrition Concerns for Aging Populations.* Nih.gov; National Academies Press (US). https://www.ncbi.nlm.nih.gov/books/NBK51837/

Intermittent fasting for weight loss: 5 tips to start. (2019, April 5). Www.medicalnewstoday.com. https://www.medicalnewstoday.com/articles/324882

Ito, S. (2019). High-intensity interval training for health benefits and care of cardiac diseases - The key to an efficient exercise protocol. *World Journal of Cardiology, 11*(7), 171–188. https://doi.org/10.4330/wjc.v11.i7.171

Johnson, A. (2018, October 14). *Mediterranean Diet Berry Breakfast Smoothie (10 Mins).* Medmunch.

https://medmunch.com/mediterranean-diet-breakfast-smoothie/

Kassel, G., & Slowiczek, L. (2018, March 30). *7 Ingredients Your Multivitamin Should Have, According to Experts*. Healthline. https://www.healthline.com/health/food-nutrition/best-vitamins-to-take-daily#4.-Zinc

Keto vs. Mediterranean: Which Diet Is Really Better for You? (n.d.). Health.com. Retrieved April 30, 2021, from https://www.health.com/nutrition/keto-mediterranean-diet

Klein, R., Rowland, M. L., & Harris, M. I. (1995). Racial/Ethnic Differences in Age-related Maculopathy. *Ophthalmology, 102*(3), 371–381. https://doi.org/10.1016/s0161-6420(95)31012-3

Knutzen, K., Brilla, L. R., & Caine, D. (1999). Validity of 1RM Prediction Equations for Older Adults. *Semantic Scholar*. https://doi.org/10.1519/1533-4287(1999)0132.0.CO;2

Livermore, S. (2020, December 7). *Indulgent Salmon Recipes for a Healthy Dose of Omega*. Delish. https://www.delish.com/cooking/g2039/salmon-recipes/

Mayo Clinic Staff. (2019). *Mediterranean Diet: A heart-healthy eating plan*. Mayo Clinic; https://www.mayoclinic.org/healthy-lifestyle/nutrition-and-healthy-eating/in-depth/mediterranean-diet/art-20047801

Mediterranean Quinoa Bowls with Roasted Red Pepper Sauce. (2015, December 21). Pinch of Yum. https://pinchofyum.com/mediterranean-quinoa-bowls-with-roasted-red-pepper-sauce

November 2006 - Volume 16 - Issue 6 : Clinical Journal of Sport Medicine. (n.d.). Journals.lww.com.

https://journals.lww.com/cjsportsmed/Abstract/2006/11000/Weight_Training_in_Youth_Growth

Nutrition Insurance Policy: A Daily Multivitamin. (2012, September 18). The Nutrition Source. https://www.hsph.harvard.edu/nutritionsource/multivitamin/

Nutrition through life - British Nutrition Foundation. (n.d.). Www.nutrition.org.uk. https://www.nutrition.org.uk/nutritionscience/life.html

OliveTomato. (2013, February 4). *Olive Oil Brownies Made with Greek Yogurt*. Olive Tomato. https://www.olivetomato.com/mediterranean-inspired-brownies-made-with-greek-yogurt-and-olive-oil/

Overview. (2018). World Bank. https://www.worldbank.org/en/topic/agriculture/overview

Pan Fried Sea Bass with Lemon Garlic Herb Sauce. (2017, August 16). Bowl of Delicious. https://www.bowlofdelicious.com/pan-fried-sea-bass-with-lemon-garlic-herb-sauce/

Petty, L. (2017, June 5). *Changes in Eating Habits Over the Years: Comparing Diets Now &...* The Hub | High Speed Training; High Speed Training. https://www.highspeedtraining.co.uk/hub/changes-in-eating-habits/

Pruitt, L. A., Jackson, R. D., Bartels, R. L., & Lehnhard, H. J. (2009). Weight-training effects on bone mineral density in early postmenopausal women. *Journal of Bone and Mineral Research*, $7(2)$, 179–185. https://doi.org/10.1002/jbmr.5650070209

Raman, R. (2017). *How Your Nutritional Needs Change as You Age*. Healthline. https://www.healthline.com/nutrition/nutritional-needs-and-aging

Reiner, M., Niermann, C., Jekauc, D., & Woll, A. (2013). Long-term health benefits of physical activity – a systematic review of longitudinal studies. *BMC Public Health, 13*(1). https://doi.org/10.1186/1471-2458-13-813

Research on intermittent fasting shows health benefits. (2020, February 27). National Institute on Aging. https://www.nia.nih.gov/news/research-intermittent-fasting-shows-health-benefits

RPI: Ave price - White fish fillets, per Kg (cod prior Feb 02) - Office for National Statistics. (n.d.). Www.ons.gov.uk. Retrieved April 30, 2021, from https://www.ons.gov.uk/economy/inflationandpriceindices/timeseries/czol/mm23

Serra Majem, L., García Alvarez, A., & Ngo de la Cruz, J. (2004). [Mediterranean Diet. Characteristics and health benefits]. *Archivos Latinoamericanos de Nutricion, 54*(2 Suppl 1), 44–51. https://pubmed.ncbi.nlm.nih.gov/15584472/

Side Effects of Switching to a Healthy Diet. (n.d.). LIVESTRONG.COM. https://www.livestrong.com/article/312225-side-effects-of-switching-to-a-healthy-diet/

Tello, M. (2018, June 26). *Intermittent fasting: Surprising update - Harvard Health Blog*. Harvard Health Blog. https://www.health.harvard.edu/blog/intermittent-fasting-surprising-update-2018062914156

The Benefits of Running vs. Walking. (2018, June 18). *The Benefits of Running vs. Walking*. Consumer Reports. https://www.consumerreports.org/exercise-fitness/benefits-of-running-vs-walking/

The Mediterranean Diet — An Up-Close Look at Its Origins in Pantelleria. (n.d.). Www.todaysdietitian.com. https://www.todaysdietitian.com/newarchives/050113p28.shtml

Trichopoulou, A., & Lagiou, P. (2009). Healthy Traditional Mediterranean Diet: An Expression of Culture, History, and Lifestyle. *Nutrition Reviews*, *55*(11), 383–389. https://doi.org/10.1111/j.1753-4887.1997.tb01578.x

Use a House Cleaning Workout to Burn More Calories Doing Chores. (n.d.). Verywell Fit. Retrieved April 30, 2021, from https://www.verywellfit.com/how-to-burn-more-calories-cleaning-house-3495596

What Happens to Your Body When You Start to Eat healthy. (2019, January 11). 20 Fit. https://www.shapescale.com/blog/health/nutrition/what-happens-when-you-start-eat-healthy/

Wholemeal savoury pancakes recipe. (n.d.). BBC Food. Retrieved April 30, 2021, from https://www.bbc.co.uk/food/recipes/wholemeal_savoury_17492

Wiginton, K. (n.d.). *Pick the Right Supplements and Vitamins*. WebMD. https://www.webmd.com/diet/features/what-vitamin-should-i-take#1

www.ingramcontent.com/pod-product-compliance
Lightning Source LLC
Chambersburg PA
CBHW071117030426
42336CB00013BA/2119